Oxford

Oxford

Studies in the history of a
university town since 1800

edited by
R. C. Whiting

Manchester University Press
Manchester and New York
Distributed exclusively in the USA and Canada by St. Martin's Press

Published by Manchester University Press
Oxford Road, Manchester M13 9PL, UK
and Room 400, 175 Fifth Avenue,
New York, NY 10010, USA

Distributed exclusively in the USA and Canada
by St. Martin's Press, Inc.,
175 Fifth Avenue, New York, NY 10010, USA

British Library Cataloguing-in-Publication Data
A catalogue record for this book is available from the British Library

Library of Congress Cataloging-in-Publication Data
Oxford: studies in the history of a university town since 1800 /
    edited by R.C. Whiting.
        p.   cm.
    Includes index.
    ISBN 0-7190-3057-9
    1. Oxford (England) – History.   2. University of Oxford – History.
    I. Whiting, R.C.
    DA690.0980895   1993   92-31628 CIP
942.5'74 – dc20

ISBN 0 7190 3057 9 *hardback*

DA
690
·098
0895
1993

Typeset in Great Britain
by Williams Graphics, Llanddulas, North Wales
Printed in Great Britain
by Biddles Ltd, Guildford and King's Lynn

Contents

Figures and tables

Figures

Tables

Acknowledgements

My principal debt of gratitude is to the contributing authors to this
volume for devoted and patient efforts on their particular chapters.
Peter Howell deserves special thanks for his help in the selection of
illustrations. Photographs were drawn from the rich collection of the
Oxfordshire Photographic Archive and are reproduced with permission
of the Centre for Oxfordshire Studies, the Central Library, Oxford.

Archivists and librarians at the Bodleian Library, the Oxford
Central Library, and the Oxfordshire County Record Office have
been particularly helpful to a number of contributors. The support
given by the painstaking scholarship in *The Victoria County History of
Oxfordshire*, especially volume four on the city edited by Alan Crossley,
is evident from the notes to a number of the chapters, but it is a
pleasure to acknowledge that substantial contribution here.

First Ray Offord and subsequently his successor Jane Carpenter
at Manchester University Press provided valuable advice and patient
support during the preparation of this volume and I am grateful to
them both.

R. C. Whiting

Introduction

The University has made Oxford a special English city. The theme running through this collection of essays is the relationship between the University and its urban setting. A number of questions naturally arise about the role of such a major institution, about its influence upon the appearance and planning of the town, about the place of university groups in local politics and society and about the degree to which academics contributed to the understanding of their town. These essays do not assume that the University's influence has been all-pervasive; rather, they inquire about boundaries as much as connections, and establish the limits as well as the extent of the University's influence upon the town.

For all its fame and familiarity, however, Oxford is not easy to classify as a university town; rather, it falls between two strikingly different interpretations. The Oxford geographer, E. W. Gilbert, asking the question 'What is a university town? Is it simply a place that possesses a university as one of its institutions or should the term be reserved for a town whose main function is that of a university?' came down decisively in favour of the latter, citing St Andrews as 'strictly the only example of a true university town'.[1] Bangor and Aberystwyth followed close behind in Gilbert's list, but Oxford failed the test, at least for the twentieth century because of the motor industry at Cowley and the way in which the central university area has been inadequately protected against people and traffic. In Gilbert's view the priority was for a university to insulate itself from dynamic urban change so as to preserve the peace required for academic reflection and intellectual exchange.[2] The university town is, in this view, the cohabitation of competing forces, and whether town is more important than university depends on economic trends and town planning.

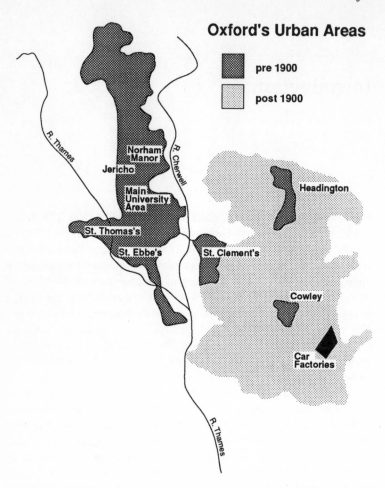

Oxford's Urban Areas

pre 1900

post 1900

1 Oxford, showing influence of geology on development, and the principal areas mentioned in the text

Oxford stumbles equally before another perspective, that of the university and the great city. While for Gilbert any encroachment upon the university by urban interests compromises the status of the university, for this other characterisation which turns upon the pervasive interaction with the city, Oxford is again a misfit. The problem here is that the town, rather than being too threatening, is too insignificant in size and status:

The Anglo-American tradition, based on the model of Oxford and Cambridge and nourished by an Anglo-American tradition of anti-urbanism is a major deviation from the central theme of the history of universities. Since their inception they have been identified with cities, sometimes second order cities, but often those great cities that dominate the political, economic and cultural life of nations.[3]

In Britain civic universities like Birmingham explicitly acknowledged this 'central theme' which was rooted in the Italian city states.[4] The intention was not simply to exist alongside other institutions but to mesh with local interests and augment the achievements of the city. By way of return, the very size of the city provided scope for academic investigation which might have general and not merely local significance.

There are many ways in which Oxford was closer to Gilbert's view of the university town than the 'city' model. Oxford certainly has had a profound impact upon national life, but this has derived from its intellectual and political activity and not from association with a city of commensurate standing. In turn, the rural aesthetic was firmly grasped by those interested in Oxford's preservation. The Oxford Preservation Trust which features in Ian Scargill's chapter placed a good deal of emphasis upon the protection of the contryside around the city, but was generally less effective at handling the urban environment. One of the complaints in Thomas Sharp's *Oxford Replanned* (1948) was the stronger attachment to rural rather than urban beauty by Oxford's enthusiasts. Sharp's criticism was not so much about the celebration of the surrounding countryside but more of the way in which the city was cluttered with rural *motifs*, from the Magdalen College rose garden at the foot of the High, to the use of certain kinds of Cotswold stone for particular buildings. In the twentieth century the controversy over protecting the city from cars turned on questions of traffic management, but it also showed the attachment to Christ Church meadow, close to the heart of the city, which its supporters claimed as a fine example of *rus in urbe*. Another viewpoint which was not an affirmation of rural values but which did, none the less, want to exclude commerce and industry, emerged in the 'twin-city' approach to Oxford's planning. The aim of this strategy was to concentrate industry and commerce at Cowley to the south-east of the city in order to regain for the university area some of the peace and quiet required for academic pursuits.

However, while the rural preferences might be well-attested, they cannot obscure the reality of involvement in the town which the essays here describe. An obvious contrast between Oxford and other 'purer' university towns lies with the region in which it was located. Oxford was situated within a prosperous and developing south-eastern region which presented the town with opportunities and choices about its character and development, in which the university had an obvious interest. The universities of Aberystwyth, Bangor, and Durham, in contrast, were not only in much smaller towns but also in regions where economic and industrial factors made a much less forceful impact. Oxford as a site for economic activity broadly defined, whether military establishments, railway undertakings or car factories, was a proposition which engaged the university in the nineteenth and twentieth centuries, and divisions of opinion ran across rather than along a town – gown divide. While an 'outsider', Thomas Sharp, pleaded for the relocation of the motor industry away from Oxford, it was a don, Henry Clay, who pointed out how foolish this suggestion was.[5] Lord Nuffield, founder of Oxford's motor industry, had difficult relations with the University, and these seem to epitomise the gulf between factory and college. Not only was there the episode of Nuffield College itself, where the devious dons added 'social' to 'science' to spoil the founder's intentions, but socially, too, there was little interaction between car executives and academics: 'There was the university: that was very much a closed shop', according to one of the directors, the gregarious Sir Miles Thomas.[6] But Nuffield himself was an awkward, reticent person even to those who mixed regularly in business circles. Sir Raymond Streat, the spokesman for the Lancashire textile industry, thought him 'the dumbest, dullest great man of the drab great men I have ever encountered'.[7] Awkward personal relations should not hide the fact that, without an heir, Nuffield gave generously to the University from one of the last substantial fortunes made from manufacturing industry.[8] Moreover, Nuffield's experience was not necessarily repeated in other examples of interaction between the University and business. The nineteenth-century experience was, as Anthony Howe shows, one of the intermingling of town and gown groups, while in the twentieth century businessmen felt the University contributed considerably to the commercial attractiveness of Oxford.[9]

The interaction of local institutions and interests was always open to modification by the role of the state. As the state extended its activities in the twentieth century, and played a decisive part in what had been more obviously private organisations, so it was to segment the components of Oxford's economy and society. The health service, education, and the motor industry came under close supervision and direction at different moments. However, Robert Waller's chapter shows how the potential for weakening the cohesion of local society was dependent upon particular policies, and that an opposite outcome was possible. In his analysis of political behaviour since 1945 he shows the health services, the motor industry, and the University showing a common interest in protecting their dependence upon certain state support threatened by the Thatcher government. The relative cohesion of Oxford institutions in the nineteenth century when the state was weak was not of necessity destroyed in the twentieth century, when the state became more extensive.

If the pressures of the wider region meant that university interests were faced with frequent stimuli for involvement in the town, it was also true that Oxford's relatively small size encouraged participation in its affairs. When Violet Butler was undertaking the research which led to *Social Conditions in Oxford* (1912) she relied upon A. J. Carlyle, the political theorist from University College, to introduce her to local trade unionists. Even with the arrival of the motor industry in force in the 1920s, Oxford remained a medium-sized town, far less complex than Birmingham, Manchester, or Leeds. For those interested in local affairs Oxford was sufficiently comprehensible to encourage intervention. Certainly, academics were never foced to retreat in the face of an overbearing urban environment, however much they may have complained about industry on the doorstep. Where universities have had to find their place in major cities, Bender has commented on 'the swing in the life of the city and the university between coherence and fragility',[10] which could never be applied to Oxford.

As the essays in this volume show, involvement was inescapable and occurred along a number of lines of connection. Voluntary service is a case in point. In the late nineteenth century there was a strong impulse nationally and within Oxford for the privileged classes to do something for the poor. A good deal of energy was expended by dons' wives in providing infant welfare on a voluntary basis to poor mothers in Oxford. But, as Liz Peretz shows, while university wives could turn their social connections to good advantage and put in many years of service, their efforts were not necessarily effective, and it was not easy to bridge the gap between the University

and the poorer sections of Oxford society. Assessing the results of
social welfare activities is not always straightforward, but merely
at the level of benefits and material provision Oxford volunteers did
less well than those elsewhere. In Tottenham the efforts springing
from an entirely different milieu – the Co-op and nonconformity
rather than the college and Anglicanism – seemed more substantial
than those made in Oxford.

Peretz's suggestion that voluntary work in Oxford benefited the
provider as much as the recipient also has echoes in the special
system of university representation on the city council, which is
featured in the chapters by Howe and Waller. As Cannan hinted,
and others practised, the University's right to nominate members
on to the council was used by some as a way of obtaining practical
political experience without the chore of electioneering.[11] Others
interpreted it differently, putting in many years of disinterested
service in the manner of Norman Chester (Nuffield) or Geoffrey
Marshall (Queen's). But university representation was never used
as a way of putting across a university view in local affairs; had it
been so, the privilege might not have lasted down to the 1970s.
Indeed, as Waller shows, this feature of local representation was
ended because of the way it seemed to favour one of the parties – the
Conservatives – rather than the University itself. It would be wrong
to assume that the University could have put together a common view
from the constituent colleges had it wished to do so, and so used
university representation to press a well-defined opinion upon the
city council. During the debates over the Oxford roads system there
was rarely a commonly-held university view, because some colleges
were more seriously affected than others by particular schemes.

If the University was slow to catch on to town planning, so that
the expansion of Cowley by the arrival of the Pressed Steel factory
in 1926 occurred without the expression of a university view, the
impact on the town through architecture and landownership was more
powerful. As Peter Howell shows, the key question for the modern
period was how far the achievements in place by the eighteenth
century could be sustained. The record of college and university
building has been uneven, but with plenty of triumphs even in the
modern period (St Catherine's College, for example). Colleges could
be both timid and inspired in their patronage; such unevenness was
probably inevitable, and becomes more excusable when professional
architects admitted that they had been overawed by the historic

setting in which their work was to be located. The town has obviously benefited from the successes in college and university building and has also provided some admirable buildings for its own use. Two adverse tendencies have been the excessive imitation of the work of university architects ('too much Jackson') and the taking over of good town buildings by the University and their use for different purposes. This, in turn, was a function of university expansion from the 1960s which put pressure on the central area and led the city council to fear that the balance between town and university was being tipped too far towards the latter.[12]

A distinctive feature of Oxford has been the high proportion of land in the city owned by the colleges. With St John's as her example, Tanis Hinchcliffe shows how a college could have a powerful impact on the appearance and social structure of residential sectors of the city. The college maintained West Oxford as a socially mixed area and also limited university expansion into the Victorian suburb of North Oxford. In this latter respect colleges as local landowners were not merely proxies for university interests, who could thereby provide a more flexible environment for university expansion than would have been possible through more conventional private land-owners; they had their own interests to pursue, and while college land was frequently sold to the University this was by no means automatic, nor were deals struck at bargain prices.

Oxford's relatively modest scale, while encouraging a university voice in its affairs and giving prominence to its buildings and land-ownership in the structure of the city, seemed necessarily to limit its interest as a subject for academic investigation. The closer it came to a university town in Gilbert's sense, the less it could represent urban features found more generally. Certainly the geological influences obstructing a concentric pattern of development and intensifying the university character of the central area meant that Oxford would always have highly idiosyncratic features from a sociological or political point of view. Although Collison and Mogey argued that their work on residential segregation would be of relevance to other English towns, the factors operating in Oxford's case – college landownership and unusual spatial development – added peculiar features. Waller's essay shows just how volatile student opinion could be when it was deployed in an Oxford constituency rather than dispersed in the students' home constituencies.

Some studies have exploited Oxford's particular characteristics without searching for any more general significance; H. E. Salter's survey of the medieval walled city which was published in the Oxford Historical Society series would be a case in point.[13] But it would be wrong to claim that Oxford has responded to academic investigation only where the particular rather than the general is at stake. It is true that there have been some kinds of study which Oxford's modest scale could not sustain; but, equally, there have been general questions for which Oxford could provide useful answers, as is shown here by the editor's chapter on the segregation of the Cowley car workers. In the 1970s Jean Gottmann found Oxford highly relevant for illustrating the role of universities in urban concentration generated by intellectual rather than material exchanges. The title of Barnett House's two-volume study *Survey of Social Services in the Oxford District* (1938 – 40) concealed a range of enquiry which went far beyond social administration to take in the dimensions of change in an expanding area. Among its authors were a number who achieved distinction in the social sciences – Russell Bretherton, Ruth Cohen, E. W. Gilbert, Robert Hall – and the work deserves fuller recognition among the social surveys of the twentieth century.[14]

Of the university population the students probably had the least impact upon the town, except in the impersonal way as consumers. Few of the students were drawn from the town or the immediate region.[15] The college was quite deliberately emphasised as the focus of intellectual and social life, and university authorities did their best to insulate undergraduates from any of the socialising effects of the town. These efforts were not completely successful and certain 'leakages' – principally in the form of drink and sex – were necessary to make the system tolerable.[16] After 1945 especially undergraduates were given more formal freedoms in the use of city pubs, for example. The substantial proportion of the undergraduates who lived outside their colleges in lodgings (around 40 per cent of undergraduates for much of the twentieth century) certainly saw more of Oxford life, but if they spent their time in Oxford pubs near to the city centre they jostled with other students rather than with the natives. Only if they were amongst the smaller number who lived some distance from the university area in, say, Cowley, did they join in a more conventional, non-university social life.[17]

These connections with the town were, however, fundamentally different in kind from those at other universities. Robert Anderson's study of Aberdeen shows how Scottish students shared with the middle class a cultural and social life centred on the town rather than on the University. Here the town provided an element of culture and broader education not found or looked for in the Oxford model.[18] It is difficult to gauge whether or not the Oxford population gained a great deal from the specific cultural contribution of the University (aside from the beauty of the buildings, that is). It is possible that the University provided an audience for cultural 'imports' which exerted a stronger attractive force than the town could have generated by itself. That the student output proved enticing to the town population may have been more doubtful. Sir Miles Thomas, who as an affluent car executive in the inter-war years enjoyed an active social life amongst the Oxford professional classes, and who regularly visited the theatre, steered clear of university productions: 'Particularly we could not get on with amateur productions of pieces like 'Peer Gynt'; which, played with great deliberation by the Oxford University Dramatic Society, went on far too far into the Sunday morning, instead of finishing crisply enough to leave an hour or so for friendly relaxation before going to bed'.[19] However, by the second half of the twentieth century student experiences began to converge, and Aberdeen's became less strikingly different from Oxford's in which middle-class social life retreated into the suburbs, leaving students to be 'faithful to an older ideal of collective, public enjoyment. In this they share the position of the young and unmarried generally, and as a result the norms of student life relate to a generational rather than a class ideal, expressed culturally in music and sartorial tastes.'[20] The marginal role of students in Oxford's recent urban history is therefore not unusual in British university experience.

Oxford contains a rich pattern of connections between the city and the University even if it is hard to categorise in the urban history of university towns. The University has had a defining role in the city's identity, and its economic, social and political activities have never suffered the eclipse they might have experienced in a larger urban environment. But the town has never been subordinate to university interests, and this balance gives Oxford its fascination, and one which the chapters in this volume try to explore.

Notes

1   E. W. Gilbert, *The University Town in England and West Germany. Marburg, Göttingen, Heidelberg and Tübingen, viewed comparatively with Oxford and Cambridge*, Chicago, 1961, pp. 2–3.

2 Gilbert, *University Town*, p. 71.

3 Thomas Bender (ed.), *The University and the City. From Medieval Origins to the Present*, Oxford, 1988, p. 3. Oxford and Cambridge do not feature in this fine collection of essays.

4 Michael Sanderson, 'English civic universities, 1870–1914', *Historical Research*, LXI, 1988, p. 95.

5 Clay was at the time Warden of Nuffield College, and his review of Sharp's book was in the *Oxford Magazine*, 24 April 1948, p. 378.

6 Miles Thomas, *Out on a Wing*, London, 1964, p. 155.

7 Marguerite Dupree (ed.), *Lancashire and Whitehall: the Diary of Sir Raymond Streat*, Manchester, 1987, vol. 2, p. 296.

8 Besides the biography by P. W. S. Andrews and Elizabeth Brunner, *The Life of Lord Nuffield. A Study in Benevolence and Enterprise*, Oxford, 1954, there is a useful short account of Nuffield's life by R. J. Overy, 'William Richard Morris', in D. Jeremy (ed.), *Dictionary of British Business Biography*, London, 1985, vol. 4, pp. 334–41.

9 Barbara Baird, 'The web of economic activities in Oxford', *Ekistics*, CCLXXIV, 1974, p. 45.

10 Bender, *University and City*, p. 4.

11 J. Redcliffe-Maud, 'Administrative studies in Oxford 1929–39', in A. H. Halsey (ed.), *Traditions of Social Policy. Essays in Honour of Violet Butler*, Oxford, 1976, pp. 74–5.

12 Oxford city library, 'Report of the city architect and planning officer on the implications of Report of Commission of Enquiry (Franks Report)', 11 October 1966, p. 3.

13 H. E. Salter, *Survey of Oxford, 2 volumes*, Oxford Historical Society, 1960 and 1969. Volume 1 was edited by W. A. Pantin, volume 2 by Pantin and W. T. Mitchell. Volume 1 contains an appreciation of Salter by Pantin. More recently Mary Prior, *Fisher Row. Fishermen, Bargemen and Canal Boatmen in Oxford 1500–1900*, Oxford, 1982, has demonstrated the value of social history at the micro-level.

14 Bretherton contributed to trade cycle theory and made a distinguished career in the civil service, as did Robert Hall (later Lord Roberthall), who headed the cabinet's economic service. For Ruth Cohen's reputation as an economist see Elizabeth and Harry Johnson, 'Ruth Cohen: a neglected contributor capital theory', in *The shadow of Keynes. Understanding Keynes, Cambridge and Keynesian Economics*, Chicago, 1978.

15 In 1960 only 6 per cent of undergraduates came from within 30 miles of the city.

16 V. H. H. Green, 'The university and social life', in L. S. Sutherland and L. G. Mitchell (eds.), *The History of the University of Oxford. Volume 5. The Eighteenth Century*, Oxford, 1986, pp. 336–8. T. H. Aston, 'Undergraduate lodgings in Oxford, 1868–1914', unpublished seminar paper.

17 Peter Knight, 'Aspiring to dream', *Wadham College Gazette*, January 1992, p. 43.

18 R. D. Anderson, *The Student Community at Aberdeen 1860 – 1939*, Aberdeen, 1988. Dr Anderson's volume is one of the excellent Quincentennial Studies in the History of the University of Aberdeen produced under the general editorship of Jennifer Carter.

19 Thomas, *Out on a Wing*, p. 149.

20 Anderson, *Student Community*, pp. 117 – 18. Some of the topics mentioned in this introduction are pursued further in my essay 'The University and locality: a transformed environment', in Brian Harrison (ed.), *A History of the University of Oxford. Volume 8. The Twentieth Century*, Oxford, forthcoming.

Intellect and civic responsibility: dons and citizens in nineteenth-century Oxford

The study of nineteenth-century towns has most often focused on conflict between classes and sects, a background against which Oxford has appeared an haven of quasi-rural stability and the bastion of the patrician lost order of England before this itself was swept away by Cowley and the motor car.[1] Before the coming of Motopolis, historians have found little evidence, in this gentlemanly urban setting, of the popular movements or class conflict of the industrial North, while in the intellectual heart of Anglicanism, nonconformity was reduced to a marginal existence.[2] But this stereotype can be carried too far. It is clear that Oxford does offer its own unique version of urban tension, that created by the coexistence of thriving market town and expanding national university. This relationship expressed itself less through classes but more through institutions, the University and the colleges often in apparent conflict with the municipal corporation and the freemen with whom the majority of Oxford's residents in some way identified. In these relations deference and economic dependence vied with the townsmens' desire for emancipation from university tutelage. At the same time, dons, for whom Oxford had in the past been primarily a *ville de passage*, now became permanent residents, ready to see themselves as 'householders' and 'citizens' as well as custodians of college and university property. Citizenship in later nineteenth-century Oxford was presented, above all by T. H. Green, as an arena in which townsmen and gownsmen could unite in pursuit of a higher goal, the recreation of the Greek *polis* in the local setting, a goal which Green's New Liberal followers would later pursue at the national level. This idealist reconciliation of the conflict between town and gown was matched at the social level by growing co-operation on practical concerns. Its success depended upon plain living as well as high thinking. For, as Beerbohm noted in decrying Oxford's lost contrasts and charm, 'The townspeople now looked like undergraduates and the dons just like townpeople.'[3] The extent to which city and university went beyond coexistence and achieved a more symbiotic relationship is the theme of this chapter.

The relationship between city and university has been surprisingly neglected for the nineteenth century. Historians of universities have been concerned above all with institutional change and syllabus reform, while the study of universities and society has concentrated on the composition of the student body, to the neglect of such equally intriguing subjects as the social origins of the dons themselves.[4] Even Engels's most interesting account of the emergence of Oxford's dons as a professional group has little to say on their part in local society.[5] This neglect is of course readily explicable in the terms of the self-image of many dons in the early and mid-nineteenth century. For some, the college curtilage defined the limits of human life.[6] For others, the town was merely a thoroughfare on the way to the metropolis, the continent, or the country house. The counties surrounding Oxford offered numerous agreeable resorts for those anxious for acceptance in, or who saw themselves as part of, county society. Warden Ashhurst of All Souls, for example, was 'taken in in every way' by Lady Frances Waldegrave at Nuneham Courtenay in the 1850s.[7] Jowett was not alone in enjoying regular retreats to Claydon Verney.[8] Blenheim remained the ambition of many and the achievement of the few.[9] County families like the Harcourts and Berties were also regular participants in university, town, and county life. But for some dons an active part in civic life was inescapable. The University's and colleges' positions as leading employers and property-holders in Oxford as well as historic privileges concerning trade and police all necessitated donnish involvement in local government. The duty to serve as street commissioner or paving trustee, especially after the Mileways Act of 1771, became almost an obligation of university and college office. These duties fell above all on the most permanent members of the University, the heads of house, at a time when most dons still expected a fellowship to be a stepping-stone to high clerical office – or at least a well-paid country living – and when celibacy was still the usual condition of academic tenure.[10] It was therefore a relatively small group of men who built up links of any substance with civic Oxford. Nevertheless, these ties were not only those of necessity but also of sentiment. Oxford provided a small group of professional, brewing, and banking families who intermingled as a cohesive and mutually acceptable local elite.[11] Interestingly, the Parsons family in the 1810s provided both a mayor and a vice-chancellor and later generations continued to move in both circles.[12] It was not unknown for heads of house to find wives from local families; for example, Mark Pattison in 1861 married Francis Strong, the daughter of the manager of the London and County Bank at Iffley.[13] This small professional bourgeoisie, drawn from town and gown, dominated early Victorian Oxford.

The town whose natural leaders they formed was, compared with many in nineteenth-century Britain, both stable and peaceful. Population growth was at its peak in the years 1821 – 31 (26 per cent, well in excess of the national rate of 14.9 per cent) but thereafter grew at more modest rates, comparable to those of towns like Bath, Chester, and Worcester.[14] In 1911, as in 1831, domestic service constituted the largest single occupational group, with 27 per cent of the total.[15] But Oxford's *ancien régime* was not wholly undisturbed by popular disorder, and rural conflict might, as in 1831, threaten to overspill into the town.[16] In 1867, Oxford also experienced some of the last bread riots in England.[17] Nor was Oxford free from traditional social threats, those of poverty and prostitution, common to many pre-industrial towns. Here were some sources of inevitable tension between town and gown. Nevertheless, national issues of religion and education preoccupied the university world in the 1840s and 1850s, while the town enjoyed the benefits of reformed government after 1835. It was therefore only slowly that there emerged any sense that university and civic ambitions might diverge, that intellect might be a force dissociated from locality, and that the interests of a 'national' university might not be identical with the material prosperity of local citizens.

I

These issues were first voiced in detail in the 1860s, when the well-known debate over the part to be played by the University in the education of the nation was complemented by a local debate over the place of the University in the economy of the city.[18] Two issues provoked a wider debate, the suggestion in 1865 that Oxford might become the site of the workshops of the Great Western Railway, and the proposal in 1872 that it might become the depot for local military forces. Both brought into the open the often implicit conflict between the welfare of the town and that of the University, between the claims of the locality and the interests of the nation.

In the first of these episodes, in 1865, university resistance was widely held to have defeated the Corporation's desire to revive Oxford's flagging economy by offering the lease of Cripley Meadow to the GWR for its new workshops. This proposal offered Oxford a prospect of industrial growth and employment half a century before the Cowley motor works finally brought industrialisation to Oxford. Here two different conceptions of Oxford as a city were brought into conflict. On the one hand, the opponents of the workshops, led incongruously perhaps by the free-trade liberal Goldwin Smith, put forward the University's national vocation as a good superior to that of the locality. Academic cities were, for Smith, a national possession, an element in national character and greatness to be cherished even more 'in proportion as the noise and smoke of manufacturing and commercial industry spread over the other cities of the land'.[19] Above all, it seemed to Smith that the moral character of Oxford constituted its claim on parents and the nation to educate youth, a character which manufacturing works would substantially undermine by bringing the evils of great cities to small towns. Smith's case was dressed up in economic garb. He thus claimed that any damage to the University would harm the town whose greatest economic good remained 'its reputation ... as a resort for the students and literary men'.[20] He also held that the forecast increase in population from the works, perhaps some 1,250, would harm Oxford's residents by pushing up house rents and food prices. For good measure, Smith also urged directors of the GWR that the site chosen was unhealthy, 'the worst in the town', and that self-interest and the national good dictated a different site. The choice of Oxford would represent a dangerous and 'artificial' distortion of the 'natural' workings of the economy.

These arguments, curious for a member of the Manchester School, perhaps reveal Smith's determination to preserve Oxford as a national good to be reformed and opened to dissenters, a struggle in which he played a leading part.[21] But they were also arguments behind which any opponents of change could respectably take cover.[22] Other arguments were also voiced. For example, James Parker resisted the prospect of thousands of unwholesome dwellings, believing that

Oxford had reached its natural (geological) limits of healthy residence, while others feared the Radcliffe Infirmary would be unable to cope with an increase in accidents and sickness, a claim denied by its registrar (also the local coroner), E. L. Hussey.[23] The works would also, it was suggested, not improve the condition of labour but merely attract more unskilled labour and vagrants to a town already suffering an excess of both. Finally, and ingeniously, it was argued that a company employing thousands would lead to the political enslavement of Oxford to a great company and the loss of its political independence so far protected from the grasp of the University. Interestingly, Smith felt compelled to urge an alternative economic prescription. He advocated the establishment of art manufactures in Oxford as more suited to the inhabitants, a proposal which fitted in well with the recent meeting to set up a School of Art in Oxford, although the aims of neither were to be successful in the long term.[24]

Nevertheless, the University as a whole was by no means united in its opposition to the railway works. It seems that the proposal originated with Thorold Rogers, Drummond Professor of Political Economy, and two dons publicly expressed far more positive, if peculiar views. Richard Greswell, for long the bastion of Gladstone's interest in the University, realised that the University could only offer limited employment to the town whose expansion of numbers was outrunning jobs created – and that in particular only Oxford's inner parishes really benefited from the University's presence. Nor did he think the University could really oppose on principle the 'Manufacturing System', having been an early advocate of steam power and child labour in order to print the Authorised Version of the Bible twenty years earlier. For Greswell the railway works promised a less demoralising form of employment for the town, offering physical and moral benefits, and a providential means of delivering the University from its discreditable work practices.[25] Charles Neate, on the other hand, as both Oxford's MP and former Drummond Professor of Political Economy, set out more directly to combat Smith's assertions, denying that Oxford's prosperity depended primarily on the University, claiming for the town the right to judge its own best interests, upholding the benefits of the works in terms of regular, skilled, and well-paid employment, and urging the opening-up of Oxford's moral influences and educational facilities to the working man. For Neate the GWR constituted 'our great modern benefactor', a nineteenth-century version of Lord Nuffield.[26]

On the whole, this was probably the view shared by most Oxford residents, although some freemen dissented.[27] Moreover it seemed even to opponents that the town's case in favour of the GWR works would prevail.[28] Nevertheless, in the autumn of 1865 Oxford's prospect of economic progress fell victim to a Board coup against Richard Potter, the chairman of the GWR. For the Oxford scheme appeared as one of several grandiose and extravagant plans which some of Potter's colleagues believed threatened the solvency of the company. Potter was replaced by Daniel Gooch, who held no brief for this scheme, and under whom a far more modest workshop expansion was undertaken at Swindon, with which Gooch was strongly identified both as former chief engineer of the GWR and as MP for Cricklade between 1865 and 1880.[29] The vagaries of tycoon politics rather than the power of scholarly or civic argument had left Oxford to its dons as an arena favourable to moral purity and aesthetic sensibility, even at the cost of its development as a great commercial or industrial centre.

Similar issues arose shortly after this affair with the proposal, under the Military Forces Localisation Act of 1872, that Oxford should become a regional centre for army recruitment and militia drilling. This suggestion, once again supported by the townsmen, was heralded by the University as a major threat to academic discipline. Hebdomadal Council set up a delegacy to watch developments, which reported strongly on the 'inconvenience of a collision between military life and academical discipline', a view reinforced by a memorial of twenty-four professors and eighty-nine dons.[30] In particular, George Rolleston, Professor of Anatomy but long active in civic life, protested against the inevitable moral harm associated with 'an assemblage of young men in the vicinity of large towns', and cast doubt on any countervailing economic benefits to the town from the presence of many but poorly-paid soldiers. He urged forward the hard facts of the Contagious Diseases Acts, although he disclaimed any prejudice against soldiers.[31] Nevertheless, the town's MPs, Cardwell in 1872 and Hall, his Tory successor in 1874, supported the scheme. Against it the University mobilised its considerable national power – with the University MPs and Chancellor, Lord Salisbury, spurred on by the Liberal Thorold Rogers, leading the parliamentary resistance.[32] Once more, at the forefront of the campaign were the needs of a national university to uphold an environment conducive to morality and decency, for 'a vice which the University is, by public opinion, and by the nature of its duties, bound to repress, is no vice, or a venial one, in the army'.[33] University opposition in this case failed.

Cardwell, both Oxford City MP and Secretary of State for War, upheld
the case for Oxford on plausible military grounds. The University
continued to believe that 'it has been probably imperilled and certainly slighted for no other apparent reason than that of two election
intrigues'.[34] Yet ironically, when the University MP Gathorne Hardy
succeeded Cardwell at the War Office in the Conservative Administration of 1874, he reluctantly completed the project of his predecessor.
Even so, the subsequent arrival of the Cowley barracks did not
wholly submerge Oxford in the expected torrent of vice and moral
turpitude. Later nineteenth-century Oxford failed to rival Berlin
in its combination of military prowess and academic virtue. But
this issue had once again brought to the forefront the conflicting
demands of a national university and the local economy.[35]

Interestingly, too, later nineteenth-century Oxford did end up
with a considerable military presence. For the 1870s also saw the
creation of the Oxford Military College (Limited), a private venture
company set up to educate the sons of officers and others for army
careers but hoping to gain the benefits of admission as unattached
students within the University.[36] Opened on 20 September 1876,
it proffered a unique blend of bodily and mental exercise, of military
and university training. Its Council included, alongside the top
brass and Tom Hughes, dons such as J. F. Bright, A. G. Butler, and
G. W. Kitchin, dean of unattached students, with Humphry Ward
its director of studies and Arthur Acland, later Secretary of State
for Education, among its instructors.[37] But the dons failed to see
eye-to-eye with the majors and this impressive line-up soon fell
apart and the dons withdrew.[38] The shareholders persisted, largely
military men, but with a sprinkling of grocers and dons, although
the college was sustained primarily by the interest of Lord Wantage
and the wealth of his father-in-law, the banker Lord Overstone.[39]
Its annual prize-giving provided a social occasion for county and
university but its career was chequered, closing finally in 1896.[40]
Even so, things military remained a growing university interest,
for the Fellows of All Souls did not disdain the playing of Kriegespielen
and, in the early twentieth century, military history gained a chair.[41]
The town reciprocated with the election as its MP in 1892 of the
Indian Army officer and author of the 'Battle of Dorking', Sir G. T.
Chesney, while his successor Viscount Valentia served with distinction
in the Boer War, a record put to good electoral use.[42]

Ironically, in resisting the idea of a military depot, one prominent don, George Rolleston, had initiated inquiries into the moral inconveniences associated with the 'assemblage of large numbers of unmarried men in a large town'.[43] Yet these 'inconveniences' were ones with which Oxford had long been familiar. For prostitution had often confronted the proctors as both the most serious threat to discipline in the University, and a source of tension with the town.[44] University police powers were extensive with regard to prostitution, having been specially protected against the terms of Peel's Vagrant Act of 1825.[45] Periodically, resentment flared as these powers were seen unduly to discipline the 'wives and daughters of citizens' rather than to repress and punish undergraduates.[46] The suspicion of some less progressive dons that the new lodging-houses in the town in the 1870s would become the inevitable source of moral delinquency was also the focus for civic resentment.[47] Nevertheless, the real conflict created by prostitution was over the cost and responsibility for its repression. By the 1890s, such responsibility fell increasingly on the city JPs rather than on the Vice-Chancellor, part of the broader resolution of conflicting authorities which characterised town – gown relations in the later nineteenth century. Even so, the Vice-Chancellor's legal powers remained a source of civic discontent, while the regulation of prostitution remained the leading disciplinary task facing the proctors, one which possibly heightened university sensitivity to threats to Oxford's moral ambience, whether from a debauched soldiery or an impoverished working class.[48]

Concern for Oxford's moral environment was succeeded in the later part of the century by a belated concern for the physical fabric of the city. The Regius Professor of Modern History in 1899 lamented what he saw as the city's ideal, 'to make the place a factory town, independent of the University', for which it was ready to pull down dozens of old buildings.[49] The colleges had themselves already engaged in this process and building in Oxford had seen little planning or preservation. Yet Powell now reported 'dozens of men anxious to keep and uphold old buildings'. Among such, Phelps of Oriel led lobbies to encourage town-planning schemes, while Mrs Toynbee rallied to the defence of Bartlemas Chapel and Field, now neglected by Oriel yet an object of beauty and good to the poor of Oxford for 700 years.[50] A. C. Headlam, a former Fellow of All Souls but now Principal of King's College, London, in 1913 interrupted his work for Christian reunion to call, with equal lack of success, for a great town-planning scheme between university and city.[51] Oxford dons faced a stymying conflict between college and *polis*, between profit and pleasure, while its geographers wrestled with the empire, not with town planning. Symptomatically, even its one effort at a 'garden suburb' at Hinksey failed to make any headway.[52]

II

The belated recognition by Oxford dons of the need for town planning was, in a way, testimony to the autonomous nature of Oxford's physical growth in the nineteenth century. As a planning body, the University lacked power outside its own property. Colleges, above all St John's, did, as landlords, influence Oxford's suburban growth.[53] Yet Oxford, like most towns, was the outgrowth of speculative building, and even developments like Park Town were investments by local men for profit, not by dons for aesthetic pleasure.[54] By 1875, the Local Board had acquired an important influence through its by-laws.[55] Such powers did not restrain or redirect building growth, but merely set minimum standards for houses to be erected. As a result, by 1900 most dons considered Oxford decidedly 'overgrown'.[56]

The autonomy of Oxford's growth was also a reflection of the town's increasing independence from the university. The debate opened in 1865 as to the dependence of the town on the university was resolved firmly in favour of its relative self-sufficiency. This was, for example, seen in its population growth, for the rate of growth of student numbers seems to have been some way behind that of total population growth by the 1880s.[57] Interestingly, too, the proportion of taxation paid by the University in 1880 compared with 1860 had fallen from 29.4 per cent to only 19.4 per cent of the combined city and University totals.[58] Of course, as a centre of consumption Oxford still depended very much on the University's seasonal demand, and colleges were still in a strong position to bargain competitively with local tradesmen. (In Oxford's bread riots of 1867, the local animosity towards the corn merchant Isaac Grubb arose in part from his selling bread more cheaply to colleges than to the public.) Certain shops, too, depended strongly on university custom. Similarly the demand for services (financial, menial and sexual) was geared very much to the university term.[59] Yet the trend, even without the railway workshops, was towards economic growth outside university demand. Oxford was fully part of the general prosperity of the South-East, clear from the 1870s, as the region became the most advanced nationally.[60] Oxford's residents included growing numbers of retired army officers, civil servants, literary and professional men and women, a society of *rentiers*, widows, and sisters who generated a buoyant local demand for services and goods, which supplemented that of the University.[61] At the same time, Oxford's native and prospering commercial and professional classes exerted their own considerable impact on employment.

Oxford's prosperity had diverse sources. Firstly, the city became the centre for specialised trades, not only printing and publishing, but also boat-building, with the arrival of Salter's, serving not only the Thames but the Empire (for example, a river steamer built in 1905 for the Baptist Missionary Society), while Lucy's metal works found a national market for its lampposts as did Cooper's for its marmalade.[62] Secondly, Oxford continued her traditional role as a regional market and county town. This meant expansion not only of brewing but of the wholesale grocery trades, extending well into the Midlands. For example, Edward Radbone, apprenticed to a local grocer in the 1850s, gradually built up a large retail business in the South Midlands, while Grimbly, Hughes was a national not merely an Oxford firm.[63] As a result, men like the grocer G. W. Cooper were able to play a part in local affairs free from the trammels of university custom which hampered the generation of Grubb and Co. Oxford before 1914 still lacked a major industry and still suffered from an excess of labour,[64] but its commercial development had been rapid, impressive, and varied. Of course the growth of the University itself was an element in all this, but there is strong case for arguing that economic change before 1914 highlighted the growing independence of the city economy from university demand.[65]

Besides their role as consumers of goods and services, Oxford dons played little part in the direction of the local economy. Goldwin Smith's preference for art manufactures, for example, seems not to have led to any constructive support for artisan production. This was in mind when the Oxford School of Art was founded, but this hope was disappointed, while Ruskin's presence in Oxford impressed an audience of dons and ladies, not the local craftsmen. The University, through its increasingly powerful Chest, might have invested in local industry, but this likewise may well have seemed an insecure base to which to tie professorial salaries. It was as an exception, not the rule, that the Clarendon Hotel was granted a mortgage in 1883.[66] This hotel remained a rather unusual example of joint investment by town and gown, for its shareholders included many dons and former dons, Matthew Arnold, Alfred Hackman, Thorold Rogers, Goldwin Smith, A. P. Stanley, Humphry Ward, and Montagu Burrows, alongside such local worthies as Charles Symonds, the livery-stable keeper, George Tester, the fishmonger, and Henry Hatch, the bootmaker.[67] Scientific expertise was also on occasion put to local uses. For example, William Buckland, Professor of Mineralogy and an enthusiast for technological advance, chaired the Oxford Gas Company on its formation in 1818.[68] It was only in the 1870s that this company drew its leading directors from the town. The Oxford Electricity Company, formed in 1892, was on the other hand almost wholly a town enterprise, although dependent upon university custom for its early success.[69] Yet if dons contributed relatively little to modern enterprise, the University had also almost wholly abandoned its part in economic regulation. For example, by the 1840s, it rarely exercised its traditional power of discommoning tradesmen. But debt between student and tradesmen remained a perennial subject of concern, encouraging some attempt at self-regulation by tradesmen.[70] Even so, by the early twentieth century the focus of concern shifted, as enlightened Christian Socialist dons had discovered disagreeable working conditions in Oxford shops. Led by the medieval political theorist, A. J. Carlyle, they sought the institution of 'fair wages', although apparently to little effect.[71] 'Exploitation' was also now exposed through the syndicalist lens, and before 1914, G. D. H. Cole and G. N. Clark had begun a campaign of behalf on striking tram workers.[72] Here was a half-way house between dons' paternalist concern with striking agricultural labourers in the 1870s and Oxford's twentieth-century tradition of donnish involvement in the history, theory, and practice of industrial relations.[73]

III

If the Oxford economy was increasingly independent of university regulation and custom, Oxford society was subject to continuous intervention from both students and dons. By the 1830s there was already a well-established network of philanthropic and cultural institutions which embodied the primarily deferential relations between Oxford's urban poor and their university benefactors. Pregnant women, the casual poor, distressed travellers, prostitutes, and sick children were all among the numerous beneficiaries of the pervasive activities of the local philanthropist, to a great extent perhaps than in any other English town. But public intervention also took the form of involvement in local government, which offered important opportunities for dons to influence local society. In many ways it is this civic participation by dons which provides the best interface between university and city. It reveals dons in many unfamiliar guises. Generations of Oxford townsmen unfamiliar with Jowett's *Aristotle*, Liddell's *Dictionary*, or Green's *Political Obligation* were to encounter municipal works of these scholarly citizens – above all in the fields of public health, poor relief, and education.

Mid-nineteenth-century Oxford was notoriously unhealthy. Beerbohm's vapours and mists were a *fin-de-siècle* echo of the long-standing concern of Oxford's elite with the problems of flooding, drainage, and death-rates. Cholera epidemics in 1832, 1849, and 1854 had stimulated among both dons and the local medical community an important debate on public health.[74] The evident dangers of cholera had also brought town and gown together in *ad hoc* measures, for example, the Mayor, William Thorp, and Vaughan Thomas in 1832.[75] They spurred on much selfless charitable work, involving characters as disparate as the Tractarian Charles Marriott, the saintly philanthropist Felicia Skene, and the orientalist and philologist Max Mueller. By the 1850s the medical community had provided a clear critique of the public health hazards of Oxford – higher than average mortality as a result of closed courts, overcrowded homes among the poor, large open drains, irregularly emptied cesspools, as well as insalubrious lodging-houses and pigsties.[76] For some, dramatic reform was unnecessary, and improvement was possible by 'simply doing what is supposed to be done'.[77] Yet increasingly doctors and dons, led by Henry Acland, saw the urgency of authoritative change – that is to say the reconstruction of local bodies, with a Board of Health to replace the existing powers divided between Paving Commissioners and Poor Law Guardians. Acland also saw the need for a change of men, wishing to replace tradesmen and small property owners, fearful of high rates and state intervention, by dons ready to seek a physically healthy as well as morally sound Oxford. Acland, son of the Devon squire Sir Thomas Acland, and Lee's Reader in Anatomy, emerged into the forefront of Oxford life on this issue – an omnipresent doctor who would not have been out of place in Renaissance Florence. He dominated a temporary Board of Health, set up in 1854, enlisting the aid of dons and citizens,

Professor Neate alongside Alderman Butler, to combat cholera. Even the kitchens of Christ Church were put at Acland's disposal to feed the sick poor.[78] Acland's own *Memoir of the Cholera in Oxford in 1854* (1856) was designed as a spur to permanent remedies, while he also kept up a useful correspondence with leading sanitary engineers like Robert Rawlinson.[79] His campaign was eventually successful with the creation of a Local Board of Health in 1864.[80] To this the University elected one-third of the members, and Acland and Dean Liddell soon emerged as its leading lights.[81] Even so they met initial antipathy among townsmen on the Board; for example, they were both excluded in 1865 from the vital drainage committee.[82] Yet Acland, although his career now took him to the highest level of national life, retained his commitment to the locality, striving to recruit 'earnest and enlightened men' to replace the 'do-nothings' on the Board. Liddell became an expert on drains, and as a result the Board became a highly successful instrument, with a new drainage system in operation by 1880, and with Oxford's death-rate soon below the national average.[83]

Acland's energy and magnetism throughout his long medical and academic career were of immense value not only to public health but also to the creation of social bonds between town and gown.[84] As a doctor, his services were freely available to the poor, and he constantly urged the expansion and consolidation of medical facilities in Oxford, whether those of the Radcliffe Infirmary or of the dispensaries.[85] In this work he found an admirable helpmate in his wife, Sarah, née Cotton, whose extensive philanthropy was powered by the deeply religious background they both shared. The Acland Home was a just memorial to a lifetime of devotion to the unhealthy and poor of Oxford. Sir Henry, of course, had his imperious side, and in particular distrusted the Ladies' Committee of the Acland Home founded in his wife's honour, yet by his retirement in 1890, his strenous labours on behalf of the city had won the broad esteem of Oxford's citizens.[86]

The question of health in Oxford required more than the introduction of proper sewers, water-closets, and dispensaries. It depended upon the wider regional problem of water supply and the drainage of the Thames Valley itself. This issue not only dominated discussion of public health in Oxford in the 1880s but threatened the whole physical appearance of Oxford as it survives today. For at the heart of schemes for improved drainage and health lay the proposal to abolish Iffley

Lock. This was part of a plan for lowering the level of the Thames from King's Weir to Sandford whereby, it was held, the danger of flooding would be reduced and the drainage of the stagnant and noxious tributaries of the Thames improved. At the centre of this neat, radical scheme lay none other than the Vice-Chancellor of the University, the Master of Balliol, Benjamin Jowett, aided, as Acland had been, by Dean Liddell.[87] The 'abolition of the floods' became a consuming passion of Jowett during his term as Vice-Chancellor (1882 – 86), disrupting his intellectual pursuits and delaying his translation of Aristotle's *Politics*.[88] This proposal, in which Liddell had long been interested, originated in a committee set up by the enlightened agriculturist Philip Pusey, which had commissioned a report into the drainage of the Thames Valley as long ago as 1853.[89] Its recommendations – the dredging of the Thames above Iffley, a new mouth to the Cherwell, and the removal of Iffley Lock, were considered by the newly-formed Thames Valley Drainage Commission, set up in 1871, and appeared nicely to combine agricultural improvement in the county with sanitary improvement in the city. The scheme won the plaudits of civil engineers and seemed to meet needs identified by informed local opinion.[90] Nevertheless, this scheme hung fire for a number of years, for the expense of the works, over and above the needs of agricultural improvement, would fall on the University and city. But it was this plan which in 1883 Jowett pushed ahead, overcoming the financial difficulties by setting in motion his own fund-raising committee, and securing promises from the University (£3,000), the town (£2,000), and the Thames Valley Conservancy Board (£1,000), as well as seeking individual promises. With this backing, the works were begun in the summer of 1883, under the personal guarantee of Jowett and Liddell to meet expenditure incurred. The summer saw the completion of the new mouth for the Cherwell ('The Vice-Chancellor's Cut'), but work was then brought to a summary halt by the belated fears of the Oxford Waterworks Company that the removal of Iffley Lock would jeopardise the town's water supply. This difficulty was circumvented by the promise of additional works to guarantee the company (£4,000 more). These growing financial needs therefore led in October 1883 to a joint University-city appeal for further funds to complete a scheme which would confer 'a great and lasting benefit on the City and University'.[91]

Importunity fathered doubt. There now began a battle over Iffley Lock comparable to that over Christ Church Meadow in the

1960s. By December 1885 a strong body of town and gown opinion had been organised in favour of the retention of Iffley Lock, led by Professor B. Price, earlier a supporter of Jowett, and by one of Liddell's truculent Christ Church colleagues, R.G. Fausett.[92] The 'retentionists', now argued that a lower water level would, in summer, jeopardise Oxford's health by exposing mud with its accumulated sewage, while buildings and boundaries along the river would suffer; so too, they claimed, would the Botanic Garden. Less radical alternative schemes were therefore put forward whereby flood waters could be effectively removed. Yet the 'incidental' arguments posed by the retentionists were, one suspects, as important as the substantive ones, namely their fear that Jowett's ruthless abolitionism would impair the picturesqueness of the river, upset its suitability for boating, and threaten the fritillaries in Christ Church Meadow.[93] Fausett, backed by this unusual alliance of aesthetes and boating men, set up his own fund to outbid Jowett. Oxford was now riven by dispute as to which scheme would be both cheaper and healthier.

Jowett and Liddell did not give in easily to what became a populist opposition campaign. They counter-attacked with a powerful array of authorities favouring their scheme – engineers, doctors, oarsmen, and German professors.[94] Local opinion was less impressed by the weighty views of Professor Pettenkofer than it was by those of the local doctor, G.W. Child. He condemned Jowett's scheme as 'a gigantic and doubtful and costly experiment at a time of almost unexampled pressure upon the resources both of institutions and individuals'. Child also effectively pointed out that the improvements already undertaken by the Local Board had substantially reduced Oxford's death-rate to one of the lowest in the country in 1884. (From 21 deaths per thousand in 1875 to 16.5 in 1884.)[95] Strong resistance in town and university therefore spelt the end of Jowett's great civic enterprise. Very reluctantly he agreed to a compromise scheme, although insisting that all subscribers should be reconsulted before any funds should be spent for anything less than the full project to which they had subscribed.[96] Had Jowett's own scheme succeeded, Oxford's appearance, if not its healthiness, would have been dramatically reshaped. But, interestingly, opposition to it revealed no simple town – gown conflict but divisions within the university and within colleges complementing divisions within city opinion itself. Such conflict within the Oxford *polis* confirmed the editor of Aristotle's *Politics* in his preference for action by an enlightened state, whose statesmen and civil servants he himself had helped form.

Jowett's pragmatic interventionism in local affairs contrasts strongly in inspiration with the platonist idealism which drew his Balliol colleague, T.H. Green, into municipal life. For Green's ethical idealism, best known for its contribution to the making of New Liberalism, involved a doctrine of citizenship applicable in local as well as national life. This is well conveyed in the portrait of Green as Mr Grey in Mrs Humphry Ward's *Robert Elsemere* (1888).[97] Unusually among dons, Mr Grey was not only to be found in Oxford in the vacations, itself a reflection of his strong connections with the town, but he had also devoted 'years to the policy of breaking down as far as possible the old venomous feud between city and university'.[98] Green's local activities do much to bear out this fictional portrait, and historians revaluing Green's notions of citizenship have rightly emphasised their local grounding.[99] Two themes dominated Green's theory and practice of citizenship in Oxford. The first, as Mrs Ward sensed, was to create personal relationships with the Oxford people, for example by home visits to the poor, escaping the confines of Common Room and Congregation.[100] Secondly, Green strove for the emancipation of the poor from deference, drink, and ignorance. Aided by working men such as Joseph Colegrove, Green set up the Liberal Hall and the British Working Man's Club in St Clement's as a temperance and educational centre.[101] Green had in 1867 supported the Oxford Reform League, and continued to oppose aristocratic and capitalist power – it was for this reason that he insisted that the Liberals should petition against bribery and corruption after the Oxford City election of 1880.[102] Yet education remained at the centre of Green's concept of politics and citizenship. In particular, the creation of a school board in Oxford in 1870 spurred on Green's search for a civic identity which would rise above sectarian issues. (Green himself easily crossed church/chapel divides acting as Treasurer of the Church of England Temperance society, but most often attending evangelical chapels on Sunday evenings.[103]) In 1870 Green spoke for the National Educational League in Oxford, and was elected to the School Board in 1874. Green's interest in the importance of education in levelling up classes also led him directly to membership of the Oxford Town Council in 1876. The only don elected to the council before 1888,[104] Green was a pillar of the North Ward Liberal Association, with enthusiatic lieutenants in young Balliol men such as Arnold Toynbee.[105] On the council, Green became the leading advocate of the Oxford High School for Boys, an attempt to open up higher education to the sons of Oxford citizens. In this way, Green believed 'odious social demarcations' could be swept away and the tone of Oxford life sweetened.[106] Education, assisted by temperance would, Green held, make possible true political freedom, the power of citizens to make the most of themselves. The equal development of the faculties of all would produce the highest good of all, locally as well as nationally. Here then the municipality as well as the state had a vital part to play in making men free to make themselves good. Green himself was well-acquainted with the civic gospel of R. W. Dale (he was a conscientious Governor of King Edward's School, Birmingham) as well as an admirer of John Bright; his Oxford experience, however, provided a practical as well as an intellectual bridge between Birmingham liberalism and the New Liberal concept of community.

Within Oxford Green's impact was wide and deep. His example and creed drew many men and women into a new scale of involvement in the Oxford community. This was the case with Toynbee in political life and C. A. Fyffe, the historian who was to stand as a Radical Liberal in the General Election of 1885; Spooner and Phelps also acknowledged the inspiration of Green in their work in the administration of the poor law in Oxford, as did Brodrick in municipal politics.[107] Not least, after Green's early death, his widow Charlotte devoted herself to a life of philanthropy inspired by her husband's ideals.[108] Green's personal influence was unique, but it should be recalled the Oxford Liberals of an earlier generation had equally upheld their duty to raise the condition of the working class and many dons continued to play an active part in Oxford society without acknowledging any direct debt to Green. For example, the brother of Green's memoirist, Thomas Nettleship, for long the chairman of the undenominational East Oxford British School, belonged to this earlier Liberal school.[109]

Among those who may in some ways be considered Green's *epigoni*, L. R. Phelps was to play a leading role in social action in Oxford from the 1880s until the 1930s: as one obituary noted: 'no prominent member of the university ... probably has ever taken so large a share in City affairs'.[110] In fact, Phelps was far less radical than his mentor and held many individualist rather than collectivist views concerning social policy. Here Green's importance was at the level of practical social action rather than intellectual conviction. During his life, Phelps devoted a vast amount of time and attention to Oxford's poorest citizens. He was from the 1880s a mainstay of Oxford's 'Five Per cent Philanthropy', the Oxford Cottage Improvement Society, a joint town–gown affair which since 1865 had tackled the question of Oxford's poor housing. Yet poor relief became Phelps's field of practical expertise, and the basis of his national influence on social policy. From the 1880s, he was active in the Oxford Charity Organisation Society (COS), becoming a Poor Law Guardian in 1880 and chairman of the Guardians in 1912. He was undoubtedly a leading influence within both at a time when they worked closely together. Phelps's own ideas were well-expressed in an early paper to the COS read at Keble College in July 1887. They centred on a clear distinction between poverty (deprivation of comforts) and pauperism (deprivation of necessities). Poverty, he believed, could and should be relieved by charity, while pauperism was the proper sphere of the Poor Law. The COS could both relieve poverty and by timely relief prevent pauperism; the Oxford Guardians thus regularly referred cases to the COS. Pauperism itself required a workhouse regime. Phelps regularly criticised the earlier conduct of the Oxford Guardians for their laxity in this respect and prided himself on the reduction of expenditure on outdoor relief. Nevertheless he did not see the workhouse as punitive but through its medical and educational resources he believed it could restore the physical and mental efficiency of labour.[111] These were strongly individualist ideas, which Phelps held for the most part with doctrinal rigidity, although his service on the Poor Law Commission of 1905–09 to some extent acted as a solvent.[112]

Yet even in Oxford, the climate of opinion surrounding poor relief was changing markedly by 1900. As early as 1887 Phelps had failed to convince Oxford's MP, A.W. Hall, of the necessity of indoor relief only.[113] Growing numbers in town and university felt that the Oxford Guardians applied the workhouse test far too harshly, that little discrimination was exercised in favour of the deserving poor and that as a result outdoor relief was minimal compared with both adjacent Headington, and cities further afield such as Leeds.[114] Phelps may have been right to argue that the nature of poverty in Oxford had not changed – in its combination of seasonal and regional features – but this provided no real ground for persisting in the rigid adherence to prescriptions for its alleviation which now appeared

outmoded. Townsmen like the tailor Zacharias and J.T. Dodd
were increasingly vociferous critics of the Phelpsian doctrine which
dominated the Guardians under the chairmanship of J.C. Wilson,
Fellow of Exeter College.[115] In 1900 this antipathy to university
influence over the Guardians led to the formation of a 'Committee
for securing in Oxford out-relief for the deserving and aged poor
in suitable cases', backed by leading townsmen like the builder
T.H. Kingerlee and local clergymen.[116] In 1902, three dons advocated
the redrawing of Poor Law boundaries, which they believed would
reduce university influence and encourage a more generous regime.[117]
Such views were also supported by the Oxford branch of the Christian
Social Union. Oxford opinion therefore neatly mirrored divided
national opinion in the Edwardian debate on poverty.[118] Even 'The
Phelper' himself seems to have modified his attitudes as a result
of the Poor Law Commission, and the members of the Oxford COS
were to accommodate themselves to Liberal welfare reforms before
1914 with a cautious, sceptical, recognition of 'this new conception
of the state ... as the great organiser of beneficence'.[119] The Poor
Law regime described by Miss C.V. Butler in 1912 therefore represented a considerable change in spirit from that of 1890s, although
Miss Butler duly acknowledged the benefits for Oxford of the strict
regime of the past.[120]

The case of Phelps and the Poor Law is itself a useful reminder
that university intervention in social action could generate antipathy
and resentment. It was not the automatic sweetener and harmoniser
of social relations which Green foresaw. Local society could not
escape the impact of national controversy. Nevertheless, dons like
Acland, Liddell, Jowett, Green, and Phelps were all self-consciously
active citizens and did contribute significantly to the shaping of
Victorian and Edwardian Oxford. It would be inaccurate to see this
participation in civic life as new – pre-reform Oxford especially drew
forth men like Parsons into town life[121] – but the later nineteenth
century did see a more intense involvement deriving from a sense
of citizenship as well as from the sense of obligation of propertied
and Christian gentlemen. As a result residents as well as vagrants
were drawn to Oxford as a model of contemporary civic virtue,
'a good place to be a citizen in', according to A.E. Coppard.[122]
Of course, Oxford constituted no social laboratory, although it did
contribute something to the formation of New Liberalism and of
social policy. C.V. Butler, too, exemplified the English tradition

of social observation, while the COS in Oxford helped shape the British tradition of social work.[123] But Oxford produced no Chicago-style school of sociology, a distinct latecomer to the Oxford academic scene. Perhaps as a city, Oxford lacked the scale of urban social problems to encourage more than an amateur approach – even someone like Phelps was no 'expert'. This underlines the fact that men like Liddell, Jowett, and Phelps participated as citizens, out of obligation to their fellow men, and not out of professional obligation, the need to practise acquired skills. Yet this citizenship had its own limits, for not only would the experts in social action arrive on the scene, but the growing specialisation of academic life reduced the desire and ability of dons to fulfil civic duties. Hence, Edwardian Oxford saw the peak of voluntary activity by dons – men like Acland or Phelps were to have few, if any, successors.[124]

IV

The previous section has highlighted the creative role of individual dons in Oxford civic life. Yet equally important for the direction of Oxford was the formal relationship between the Univesity and the municipality. Here the later nineteenth century saw the progressive assertion of the independence of the town from university influence which had been pervasive in the early part of the century. For although Oxford had its municipal corporation, even after 1835 this lacked real power, and local government was concentrated in non-municipal authorities, such as the Paving Commissioners, where university influence was strong. The subordination of the town was symbolically rehearsed in the annual St Scholastica's Day ceremony, and it was only in 1857 that the Quaker Grubb set out to throw off this remnant of civic servitude.[125] As late as 1848, the Vice-Chancellor saw an important part of his duties as maintaining the town in due social subordination.[126] The powers of the Vice-Chancellor continued to irk not only prostitutes but also playgoers.[127] The main conflicts between town and gown in nineteenth-century Oxford however did not take the form of the set battles which tradition stressed,[128] but were above all conflicts of jurisdiction concerning police, the Poor Law, rating, paving, and health. These conflicts were pro-gressively resolved and the Local Government Act of 1888 provided the local constitutional basis for the lasting reconciliation of town and gown.

Exceptionally, one arena of local power had been dominated by the town in the early nineteenth century, that of poor relief. Under the Act of 1771 poor relief was in the hands of the parishes, and it was as late as 1844 before the New Poor Law of 1834 was extended to Oxford.[129] Under both acts, the University was exempt from the poor rate. Yet pressure for university inclusion grew from two directions. Firstly, the Oxford Guardians in the 1840s were widely considered to be unbusinesslike and drawn from the less wealthy citizens.[130] Opening up the pool of university talent was therefore attractive, even if some evangelicals in the town feared a university (high church) presence within the Guardians. But secondly, financial necessity impelled the town towards a university contribution and university representation. This the University strongly resisted, denying any legal obligation, and asserting that the University contributed the prosperity of the town in other ways.[131] This stance incurred considerable odium,[132] and eventually the University accepted the terms of the Oxford Poor Rate Act of 1854. Under this Act it elected one-third of the Guardians and was to be rated proportionately after the valuation of its property, a proportion eventually also settled at one-third.[133] Interestingly, it was this Act which Phelps later saw as ending university isolation from civic affairs.[134]

Even so, as the University faced liability for the Poor Rate, it simultaneously sought to reduce its contribution to the rates of the Paving Commission, the premier local authority in Oxford. This body had been set up in 1771, largely on the initiative of the University which had enjoyed strong representation and influence, although by the 1830s university interest had receded and townsmen played a greater role.[135] The University now held that its property represented a declining proportion of rateable property, and should now pay only one-sixth, not two-fifths of the total, a claim somewhat at variance with the argument urged on other occasions, that the wealth of the town depended upon that of the University. After various attempts to reassess university liability to this rate, its contribution was in 1848 reduced to one-third of the total, the basis for the Poor Law contribution in 1854.[136]

A decade later the future of the Paving Commission itself was at issue. As we have seen above, fears over Oxford's provisions for public health pointed to the inadequacy of the existing paving acts and the case for a new local act or the adoption of national legislation was strong.[137] Yet any new authority raised the vexed issue of the proportionate town/gown shares of representation and finance. A new bill supported by the University in 1848 was rejected by the town as an attack on municipal liberty, although the Public Health Act of 1858 proved more acceptable to local opinion.[138] Under the aegis of this Act, the Oriel don and Oxford MP Charles Neate negotiated a *modus vivendi* dividing power and liability according to the now standard ratio of one to two. But apparently, late in the day, the University went back on this and sought a division of representation of 16:21. The resulting controversy neatly illustrated contemporary ideas respecting the allocation of power between town and gown. For some, unequal university representation was justifiable as a matter of privilege and favour. Others, including Neate himself, saw the work of the Board as 'citizen's work' in which the University should expect to play a lesser part. Interestingly, where Green later saw the dons' importance as citizens, Neate tended to a more old-fashioned view that dons were not citizens, merely members of a national university: 'Oxford', he urged, 'is not our home.'[139] Neate helped solidify civic opposition to the University on this occasion, and the town councillors stood firm in their demand for a two-thirds share.[140] This was in effect recognised when after much delay, the Local Board of Health was set up in 1864, with sixteen seats each going to the University, the parishes, and the municipal corporation.[141] Yet as indicated above, despite Neate's assumptions, the work of this Board turned out to be very much dons' work in the sense that men like Liddell in the 1860s and McGrath of Queen's later in the century were highly influential within it. On the other hand, citizens were always the more diligent attenders: most dons were not yet ready to follow Green in spending vacations in Oxford.[142]

The Local Board retained its primacy in local life until 1889, for example its budget was roughly three times as great as that of the local council. Hence university activity on the Board to some extent balanced the absence of dons, with the exception of Green, from the town council. This had been low in esteem in the 1830s, although as it acquired growing responsibilities, so its standing rose. For example in 1869 it took over the main police powers of the town hitherto divided between town and gown, but now to be jointly financed and administered.[143] Yet by comparison with other towns, Oxford was distinctly slow to unite local powers under one authority. This came about only as a result of the Local Government Act of 1888 which prompted Oxford citizens to seek county borough status and the amalgamation of local authorities. There once more arose in acute form the perennial problem of the degree of university participation in civic life producing a novel solution which survived until 1974.

By the 1880s, Oxford politics had produced a new generation of substantial citizens – the corporation reflected the growing wealth and independence of the local middle class, with mayors like Walter Gray and Robert Buckell of lasting fame and impact.[144] The demand for county borough status reflected in turn their own growing civic consciousness, and their sense of Oxford's importance – as a rapidly expanding town, the seat of an ancient corporation, and of an illustrious university: as the Town Clerk urged: 'if places like some Lancashire towns which have grown up to a population of 50000 within a generation or two are to be County Boroughs, surely Oxford which has had the fullest local government for centuries ... which is a City, a Quarter Sessions, Borough and a University is entitled to this measure of local autonomy'.[145] Oxford's case for county borough status was at first turned down – it was below the minimum population of 50,000. Still, subject to the extension of boundaries, the Local Government Board agreed that the town had a 'strong case' and the key obstacle to success lay in reconciling university and civic interests.[146] This required careful negotiation between town and gown, which resulted in September 1888 in a provisional agreement whereby the University would have its own members on the council, the Local Board would be superseded, and the Council take over the full cost of policing in Oxford.[147]

This agreement met opposition in both city and university. Within the Council the Conservative Bacon noted that many influential citizens believed that the University, as a corporation, should play no part in a popularly elected body. On the other hand, he recognised the advantages in overcoming the system of duopoly and for him the sticking point was the cost of policing. He regarded it as unfair that the town should pay to police the University, a 'national property', not a local or civic one, once more turning against the University an argument previously deployed by dons against the town. More narrowly, city acceptance of this agreement turned on whether councillor–dons should take part in the election of city aldermen. Councillor Hugh Hall opposed this on the broad ground that council affairs primarily involved the working-men of Oxford. Ninety-nine per cent of dons' interests were, he believed, dealt with elsewhere, but the whole of the interest of the working classes rested in council hands. Even so university representation found general support. This rested on the desire to set aside old rivalries, an appreciation of the contribution which the University and its dons already made to local welfare, and a rejection of the idea that dons were in any way hostile to working-class interests. Some Liberals even held that if university representation helped play down the importance of party on the Council, this would be to the advantage of working men.[148]

On the university side, debate was less intense (it was the Long Vacation). Most of those involved in negotiations were content to exploit to the University's advantage the city's keen wish for county borough status. The strongest resistance came from J.C. Wilson, former chairman of the Local Board, who upheld what he saw as its superior benefits to those offered by the new authority. He opposed the University's accepting the status of a ward within the new borough and criticised the terms negotiated by Hebdomadal Council.[149] In private, Wilson canvassed the Local Government Board, deprecating what he saw as excessive financial concessions to the town, and lamenting that twelve dons among sixty councillors would be too few to achieve the desirable ending of party influence on the Council.[150] He wrote as a Conservative but disliked party in municipal affairs. Others, for example, the Master of Balliol, sympathised with the case for more councillors, but ultimately the University accepted what they saw as 'a very strong feeling' in favour of the arrangement – with a university ward (nine councillors and three aldermen), no special contribution to police costs, and the cession of licence fees to the council.[151] This was a reasonable accommodation between university privilege and civic pride. It provided a lasting framework for the practice of citizenship on the basis of the co-operation between town and gown which Green had striven for in first joining the Council in 1876.

It is therefore briefly worth considering the impact of university councillors within this highly unusual arrangement. In one way, the dons' scope for influence was limited by the continuation of a cross-party, rather than a non-party, consensus which dominated Oxford from the 1880s. In the Oxford of Buckell and Gray, the civic aspirations of dons were held firmly in check – the first university mayor thus came only with Sherwood in 1913. Dons also remained less regular attenders than townsmen – between 1897 and 1898 they averaged 10.4 meetings to 13.7.[152] Dons elected to the Council also came disproportionately from the ranks of bursars, who tended perhaps to view their civic duties in a narrow light. Nevertheless, the dons offered to the Council both specialist skills and human variety. For example, they included the economist (but also historian of local rates) Edwin Cannan, and T.L. Bullock, a man of noted administrative skills, for long British Consul in China but who, having retired to Oxford, now found himself as its Professor of Chinese.[153] Cannan perhaps above all illustrates the fruitful interaction of don and citizen. In a letter worth quoting at length, he informed his American colleague, E.A.R. Seligman:

The University elects one fifth of the City Council and have recently chosen me as one of its representatives. I find that the contemplation of local government from the inside is a thing quite worth spending few hours a week over, and perhaps in a year or two may have some thing to say about it. Unfortunately I don't feel justified in letting things go wrong in order that I may see how it is done and violent interference with the phenomena rather destroys their value for the scientific observer. At present I am trying hard to prevent a tramway 'franchise', as you would call it (we have no convenient name), which I say is worth £2,000 per annum from being given away for £200 per annum and I feel that my intervention with stores of information garnered in the Bodleian is decidedly abnormal. If I am not a deus ex machina the tramway company certainly regards me as a diabolo ex machina. There is also the difficulty about speaking frankly about a small body of which one is a member. However, there is a good deal which could be said, I think.[154]

Not all dons combined, as Cannan did, professional expertise and civic duty, yet many notable Oxford figures were ready to serve. They included the arch-Conservative detester of attendance at boards and meetings, A.D. Godley, the historian of Oriel and translator of Dante, C.L. Shadwell, and one of the strongest of the many claimants to the title of the 'last of the Oxford eccentrics', the Warden of Merton, Thomas Bowman.[155] For many dons who fitted uneasily into the new world of specialist teaching and research, the Council offered an additional sphere in which to contribute to the community with which they now identified by lifetime residence.[156] Other dons, too, used their presence on the Council consciously to build up good feeling between town and gown, for example, an earlier Warden of Merton, Brodrick.[157] Yet by 1900, Oxford produced sufficient of its own active, well-qualified citizens so as by no means to depend on donnish leadership, while for most dons the Council remained a temporary diversion from academic tasks.

The reconciliation of town and gown and the emergence of many bipartisan policies did not, however, remove all controversy from municipal life. Above all, Edwardian Oxford was to be wholly riven upon the perennially divisive issue of transport. This was no simple town – gown affair, rather it illuminates, as did the controversy over the GWR workshops, the cross-currents within town and gown. Before 1914 Oxford depended for public transport almost wholly upon horse-drawn trams, under private ownership.[158] Yet this was the age of municipal ownership and in 1897 the Council took powers to buy the trams, although delaying the application of those powers for ten years.[159] In 1905 the Council, under strong pressure, agreed not only to exercise its right to buy the tramway monopoly but to electrify the trams in the face of prospective competition from motor coaches.[160] Among university councillors, G. E. Baker, for example, was strongly hostile to municipalisation, but Cannan, supported from outside the Council by Carlyle, was in favour.[161] Cannan regarded motor-bus schemes as 'chimerical'. He gained considerable university support, with buses widely seen as smelly, dusty, and noisy. But the council scheme was hotly contested locally, both by opponents of municipal enterprise and by opponents of electrification, which townsmen like the photographer Henry Taunt believed would ruin the appearance of Oxford. They found a ready-made alternative therefore in the motor buses which William Morris was eager to run; he became the centre of the 'motor bus party', 'the vehicles of the future school'.[162] In the event the Oxford bill for electrification was passed in parliament but a local referendum denied the Council the power to run the trams.[163] They were, therefore, subcontracted to the National Electrical Construction Co., which formed a new Oxford Tramway Co., a syndicate which included few local men. By 1913 this company had failed to electrify and its management was assailed as 'scandalous'. Oxford's travellers, as well as her tramworkers, were in a state of revolt, adding consumer protest to the pre-war wave of industrial unrest, to which the dons lent a syndicalist tinge, as we have seen above.[164] The tramworker's strike failed in May 1913 but the passenger revolt succeeded – with the aid of capitalism. For William Morris launched an unlicensed, free motor-bus service, much to the chagrin of the tramway company and the Council. This broke the circle – the tramway company now abandoned electrification and the Council accepted motor buses, run by the tramway company. They have dominated the

streets of Oxford ever since – even more noisy, smelly, and dirty
in the 1990s than Cannan had predicted in the 1900s. But here
was an instructive exercise in local democracy – a lasting solution
imposed from outside the Council and irrespective of the best opinions
of university and city.

V

The diarchy which ended in municipal government in 1889 persisted
much longer in parliamentary politics, with the university seat surviving
alongside that of the city (two seats until 1885) until 1949. Within
this arrangement, while the university seat was self-contained, no
self-denying ordinance restricted donnish participation in the Oxford
constituency. Moreover, while relatively few dons were qualified as
borough voters before 1885, the university presence in political
life was marked and persistent. Above all, most candidates had
university links by education, marriage or profession. For example,
D. Maclean in 1835 was Fellow of University College, William Erle
in 1837 both Fellow of New College and son-in-law of its Warden;
Cardwell in 1853 Fellow of Balliol, while J.W. Chitty in 1880 was
Fellow of Exeter, captain of cricket, stroke in three Boat Race victories,
and Boat Race umpire. Certainly the dominant Liberal interest in
the town valued its university links. Above all, Charles Neate con-
structed a popular alliance with Oxford's artisans and tradesmen.[165]
This strong link between enlightened dons and self-respecting artisans
survived until 1867, at which point many dons saw it as ripe for
extension to the nation as a whole.[166] Nevertheless, the extended
electorate after 1867 revealed the limits to working-class emancipation.
As we have seen in the study of Green above, dependence on candidates
for jobs, the strength of the drink interest in Oxford, the link between
the freemen and venality, all provided continuing elements of corruption
within Oxford as a result of which both Tories and Liberals were to
be unseated.[167] But dons remained a leading influence within the
Liberal party before 1914 – men like A. Sidgwick behind the scenes,
and to the fore as candidates C.A. Fyffe in 1885 and a former Fellow
of New College, J. Fischer-Williams in December 1910.[168] Local
men emerged only exceptionally as candidates – for example, the
Congregationalist builder, T.H. Kingerlee, in 1895. Yet by then
Oxford Liberalism was in steep decline, with candidates hard to
find and funds difficult to raise.[169]

By the early twentieth century, Oxford had become an impregnable Tory bastion, with a string of MPs, the local brewer, A.W. Hall (1874 – 80 and 1885 – 92), the Indian Army officer and novelist G.T. Chesney (1892 – 95), and more lastingly, Viscount Valentia (1895 – 1918), reviving a family tie with Oxford from the early nineteenth century. This Tory revival depended on determined organisation among the local stalwarts, especially by the lawyers Dayman and Walsh, but the University also produced key wire-pullers. The chief of these was the Chichele Professor of Modern History, Montagu Burrows, a former naval officer, who set out to break the Liberal stranglehold on Oxford.[170] He initiated a strong Church *ralliment* on the School Board in 1870, and thereafter, with his town allies and a stream of recruits among the young Fellows of All Souls, like Charles Oman and R. L. Poole, Burrows nourished the cause.[171] Not only did North Oxford provide natural 'Villa Tories', but local Conservatism benefited substantially from the drift of the intelligentsia towards Unionism after 1886. Dons like Anson and Dicey, pillars of Unionism nationally, felt that this cause was sufficiently vital to overcome their own earlier antipathy to involvement in local politics. As a result, it has been claimed that Unionism in Oxford was second in intensity only to that of Birmingham.[172] Certain colleges now notoriously displayed party colours, while it was not unknown for college officers to deter Liberal displays by threats of eviction.[173] But the University itself lacked any clear impact on elections – it was unusual that in 1837 it was claimed that the University had intimidated policemen and shopkeepers and organised all college servants to vote for the Tory candidate.[174] Such threats were clearly unnecessary by the twentieth century, and even in the Liberal landslide of 1906, the Tory alliance held firm even after free trade had revitalised the alliance of dons and working men (and interestingly, had won over the former Tory MP, Hall[175]). Nor was the further emancipation of the working classes in 1918 greatly to benefit the party of progress in Oxford.[176] Even so, with the battles over the Union and free trade, it could at least be said that national issues had belatedly arrived on the Oxford political scene. Organisation, ideology, and deference had nevertheless sustained a solid Conservative hegemony in a town where the extensive philanthropic activities of the dons perhaps made legislative change appear less urgent than in many cities as a solution to pressing social needs.[177]

VI

The Conservative dominance of Oxford was an important part of its Edwardian image as a bastion of patrician stability, where Beerbohm could truly feel 'the gods of retrogression' ruled.[178] Interestingly, this was an image which dons and townsmen were happy to cultivate. In an Oxford marked by considerable economic growth but also extensive poverty and some industrial unrest, the image of a timeless, traditional Oxford appealed to don and working man, left and right, undergraduate and professor. The public face of Edwardian Oxford was one which sought out its Oxford story in the realms of chivalry and romance, a local 'invention of tradition' which had a pervasive effect on local culture and society. Two events marked this development. First, the Oxford Pageant of 1907 staged by Frank Lascelles, the 'modern Orpheus', provided a spectacular review of Oxford's past, a stimulus to local patriotism and civic good fellowship bringing together town and gown. As the President of Magdalen noted, 'it educated the whole community and made Oxford realize itself'.[179] Other voices failed to discern any educational or economic value.[180] Yet a reinvigorated local pride sustained a second collective festivity five years later, with the celebration of the Millenary of Alfredian Oxford in 1912.[181] This Millenary was peculiarly apt for civic celebration, for it evoked an Oxford past before any suggestion of a university. Here was a reminder to the dons that the town had an existence independent of the University which had for so long paraded its own importance to the city.[182] On this occasion, a series of lectures and exhibitions culminated in day of pageant and procession. The tone was more uplifting than half a decade ago, the emphasis less on 'gay cavaliers on prancing horses' and more on a heightened, even progressive sense of civic responsibility.[183] Due recognition was belatedly given to the independent yet interrelated existence of town and gown, an affirmation of a shared civic identity, all the more ironic as the bonding image of traditional, historic Oxford was about to be shattered for ever by Morris and the motor car.

This pageantry also interestingly accorded a full symbolic recognition of the importance of women in Edwardian Oxford. For all commentators – from Gladstone to Beerbohm – agreed that (before the motor car) the most significant change in the face of Oxford was the arrival of women from the 1870s.[184] To some this represented a threat to culture and celibacy.[185] But the pageants of 1907 and 1912, even if they in part revived a long tradition of male frivolity, also confirmed the indispensability of women in Oxford's past and present. Women in Oxford had arrived on the scene not only as students but as sisters, mothers, novelists, poets and, most unsettlingly, wives. Not only were public lectures colonised by female audiences,[186] but bachelors' walks were threatened by infernal machines, perambulators. But most markedly of all, the old age of stuffy dinner parties and ancient social decorum, if not fully extinguished, gave way to a tremendous transfer of feminine energy, time, and talent into charitable activity.[187] The wives and daughters of dons were ubiquitous in philanthropic Oxford – setting up friendly societies for working women, organising 'Duty and Discipline' movements, defending the claims of the poor, investigating social conditions, and even entering political life. As dons increasingly felt the pressures of teaching and research, voluntary work was taken up by their wives and daughters to a quite remarkable extent. This produced resentment in some quarters, but also maintained the social ligatures which underpinned the stability of pre-war Oxford.[188] Such a role was not new in kind but new in scale and intensity – few indeed were the poor who could evade Miss Butler's card index. It fell then ultimately to women to uphold the marriage of intellect and civic responsibility which Green had sought and which had marked nineteenth-century Oxford to such a considerable extent. Even so, by 1914 there were already building up the forces, those of industrial change and academic specialisation, of war and the power of the state, which would soon precipitate a permanent separation.

Notes

1   J. Morris, *Oxford*, Oxford, 1978, p. 30; M. Beerbohm, *Zuleika Dobson*, 1911, Harmondsworth, 1971; R. Whiting, *The View from Cowley*, Oxford, 1983.

2   R. Fasnacht, *A History of the City of Oxford*, Oxford, 1954; *Victoria County History, Oxfordshire* (*VCH*), vol. 4, *The City of Oxford*, 1979.

3   'Diminuendo', in *The Works of Max Beerbohm*, London, 1896, p. 152.

4   *Inter alia*, R. N. Soffer, 'The modern university and national values, 1850–1930', *Historical Research*, LX, 1987, pp. 166–87; P. Slee, *Learning and a liberal education: the study of modern history in the universities of Oxford, Cambridge and Manchester, 1800–1914*, Manchester, 1986; L. Stone (ed.), *The University in Society*, Princeton, NJ, 1974. The forthcoming *History of the University of Oxford: The Nineteenth Century* may offer a fuller view.

5 A.J. Engel, *From Clergyman to Don: The Rise of the Academic Profession in Nineteenth Century Oxford*, Oxford, 1983.

6 Even late in the century Strachan-Davidson of Balliol stressed the need for total dedication to the '*augustum commilitium*'. J.W. Mackail, *James Leigh Strachan-Davidson*, London, 1925, pp. 55–6.

7 O.W. Hewitt (ed.), '. . . *And Mr Fortescue*': *a selection from the Diaries from 1851 to 1861 of Chichester Fortescue, Lord Carlingford, KP*, London, 1958, 27 August 1852.

8 Bodleian Library (Bodl.) Ms Top Oxon b. 164. Sir Edmund Verney to William Tuckwell, 18 January 1908, recalling visits by Pattison, Mueller, and Acland. Interleaved in Tuckwell's *Reminiscences of Oxford*, 1900–13, f. 567–79.

9 J.A.R. Marriott, *Memories of Four Score Years*, London, 1946, p. 83.

10 Engel, *Don*, Appendix 1, p. 286; A. Haig, *The Victorian Clergy*, London, 1984, pp. 277–82.

11 *VCH*, pp. 184–5.

12 J. Wells, *Oxford and its Colleges*, London, 1897 (6th ed. 1904), p. 66; Bodl. Ms Top Oxon c. 828 Parsons Papers, misc; c. 835 Diary of John Parsons, 1840s, 1850s.

13 V.H.H. Green, *Love in a Cool Climate: the Letters of Mark Pattison and Meta Bradley 1879–1884*, Oxford, 1985, pp. 14–15.

14 *VCH*, p. 182.

15 Whiting, *Cowley*, p. 7.

16 The Queen Caroline Affair in 1820 fomented town–gown disturbances, as did Reform in 1830/31. W.R. Ward, *Victorian Oxford*, London, 1965, pp. 42, 77–8; C.H.O. Daniel (ed.), *Our Memories. Shadows of Old Oxford*, Oxford, 1893, p. 107.

17 See below, p. 20.

18 For the national debate, see C. Harvie, *The Lights of Liberalism: University Liberals and the Challenge of Democracy, 1860–86*, London, 1976.

19 Goldwin Smith, *The Great Western Railway Factories and Oxford. A Letter to the Editor of the 'Daily News', 1 June 1865* (1865). Smith was the son of a former director of the GWR.

20 Smith, *The Great Western Railway Factories*.

21 E. Wallace, *Goldwin Smith: Victorian Liberal*, Toronto, 1957.

22 Public Record Office (PRO) RAIL 250/129 J.P. Lightfoot, Vice-Chancellor, to R. Potter, chairman of GWR, 29 June 1865, summary of university objections.

23 James Parker, *The 'Great Western' Invasion of Oxford* (7 June 1865); A Member of Convocation, *The Proposed Removal of the Great Western Railway Works to Oxford* (27 June 1865); E.L. Hussey, *The Great Western Railway and the Radcliffe Infirmary* (20 June 1865). See too PRO RAIL 253/129 Revd E. Evans (Pembroke), J. Macbride (Principal of St Mary's Hall) to Potter, 6 and 7 June 1865 respectively.

24 Smith, *The Great Western Railway Factories* (14 October 1865).

25 Greswell, *Oxford and the GWR Carriage Manufacture* (16 June 1865); for private lobbying, Greswell to Potter, 21, 28 June, 7 July, 16 August 1865; to D. Gooch, 28 March 1866. Greswell's interest in this matter was keenly influenced by his own attempts to improve the drainage of Port Meadow, on which he spent thousands of pounds in the 1860s, but to the benefits of which he found the town oddly unappreciative. See Greswell, *Improvements in Port Meadow*, Oxford, 1863. For a personal sketch, see J. W. Burgon, *Lives of Twelve Good Men*, 2 vols., London, 1888.

26 C. Neate, *The Great Western Railway Factories and Oxford*, London, 1865. PRO RAIL 253/129 Neate to Potter, 12, 16 June 1865; RAIL 253/130 Neale to Potter 6 July 1865.

27 PRO RAIL 253/129 and 130 J. Hughes (mayor) to Potter, *passim*; 'Plebeian', *The GWR Workmen and Oxford* (7 June 1865); Anon., *Great Western Railway Works or City versus University* (9 June 1865); G. P. Hester (Town Clerk), *The GWR Works at Oxford* (20 February 1866); 'A Citizen', *Reply to Hester* (24 February 1866).

28 PRO RAIL 253/130 Liddell to Potter, 8 July; Smith to Potter, 9 July (bis) 1865, for negotiation of the terms, especially with regard to police costs, on which the company would expand at Oxford.

29 PRO RAIL 250/20, 21 GWR Board minutes, 1864–68; R. B. Wilson (ed.), *Sir Daniel Gooch: Memoirs and Diaries*, Newton Abbot, 1972), pp. 96, 108–12; A. Platt, *The Life and Times of Sir Daniel Gooch*, Gloucester, 1987, p. 151.

30 Bodl. University Archives, Minutes of Hebdomadal Council (WP [γ]/ 27/1 15 April, 10 June 1872); *The Military Centre at Oxford* (printed statement of Delegacy, 15 June 1874; for drafts of petition and statement, University Archives MR/3/4/9 23 April, 14 June 1874).

31 Rolleston, *On the Establishment of a Military Centre at Oxford* (5 July 1873); for Rolleston, *DNB*; E. B. Poulton, *John Viriamu Jones and other Oxford Memories*, London, 1911, ch. viii; W. H. Flower, *Essays on Museums*, London, 1898, pp. 357–62.

32 Bodl. Thorold Rogers Papers, Salisbury to Rogers, 18 June 1872; see too A. Beresford Hope to Rogers, 23 May 1874; N. E. Johnson (ed.), *The Diary of Gathorne-Hardy, later Lord Cranbrook, 1866–1892: a Political Selection*, 1981, 9 May, 16 July 1872, 25 May, 10 June 1873, 31 March, 22 and 23 May 1874; *Hansard, Third series*, 1872–74.

33 *Military Centre* University statement.

34 University Archives, draft statement, 4 June 1874.

35 Interestingly this was one of the themes of Ruskin's 'Meditative Dinners' in the autumn of 1874. J. Evans and J. H. Whitehouse (eds.), *The Diaries of John Ruskin*, 3 vols., Oxford, 1959, iii, pp. 827–8. But according to G. W. Kitchin, 'their *mouton aux navets* did not attract the Oxford don more than once'. *Ruskin at Oxford*, London, 1904, p. 43.

36 PRO BT 31/2183/10211 Oxford Military College Ltd. Wound up 26 July 1893; BT 31/5674/39620 Oxford Military College Ltd. Wound up 23 November 1896; New College, Oxford, Copy Letterbooks of J.E. Sewell (Vice-Chancellor), Sewell to Major Graham, 18 and 22 November 1875.

37 Bodl. *Oxford Military College*, prospectuses, 1876, 1877 and reports, 1880, 1885; Anne Acland, *A Devon Family: the Story of the Aclands*, London, 1981, p. 115.

38 Bodl. Acland Papers, Eng. Lett. *d.*81 Cyril Ransome to A. Acland, 18 February 1877.

39 Harriet S. Loyd, *Lord Wantage, V.C., K.C.B.*, London, 1908, p. 295.

40 G.B. Grundy, elected a Fellow of Corpus in 1903, had earlier presided over its death-throes. G.B. Grundy, *Fifty-Five Years at Oxford*, London, 1945, pp. 81–5.

41 Oman, *Victorian Oxford*, p. 108.

42 Bodl. election ephemera, 1900.

43 Rolleston, *Military Centre*.

44 A.J. Engel, ' "Immoral intentions": the University of Oxford and the problem of prostitution, 1827–1914', *Victorian Studies*, Autumn 1979, pp. 79–107.

45 Ward, *Oxford*, pp. 48–9.

46 'The sins of Our cities. II Oxford', *The Modern Review*, 4 January 1893, pp. 329–39.

47 Ward, *Oxford*, p. 270.

48 G.C. Brodrick, *Memories and Impressions, 1831–1900*, London 1900, pp. 384ff.; R. Buckell, 'Civic life of Oxford', *Oxford Times*, 3 May 1912, p. 12.

49 F. York Powell to S.J. Cockerell, 20 November 1899, in O. Elton, *Frederick York Powell: A Life*, 2 vols., Oxford, 1906, i, pp. 273–4.

50 Mrs C.M. Toynbee, *Bartlemas Field*, 5 March 1908. Treasurer of Lady Margaret Hall, Poor Law Guardian, sound and devout Anglican, and with a keen interest in the welfare of all.

51 R.D.C. Jasper, *Arthur Cayley Headlam: life and letters of a bishop*, London, 1960; *Burlington Magazine*, vol. 24, 1913, pp. 16–23.

52 'Garden Suburb', *c.* 1906 in Bodl. G.A. Oxon. 250 (iv); Bodl. Ms DD Harcourt *c.* 298. North Hinksey Estate papers, *c.* 1870–91.

53 M. Graham, 'The Suburbs of Victorian Oxford: Growth in a Pre-Industrial City', Leicester University Ph.D. thesis, 1985, esp. pp. 146ff. See also Hinchcliffe, below, *passim*.

54 PRO BT 31/289/996 Park Town Estate Co. Its records are in the Bodleian Library.

55 Graham, The Suburbs', pp. 95, 173ff.

56 E.g. J. Wells, *Oxford and its Colleges*, London 1897 (2nd ed. 1904), p. 13.

57 Engel, *Don*, p. 291, for student numbers, *VCH*, p. 182, for population.

58 Income Tax assessments for Schedules A, B, D, for 1859–60: *Parliamentary Papers, 1860, XXXIX, pt. II*; Income Tax assessments for Schedules A, B, D, E, for 1879–80, *Parliamentary Papers, 1882, LII*.

59 C. V. Butler's *Social Conditions in Oxford*, London, 1912, paid especial attention to the University's impact on unemployment, the neglect of which she felt 'particularly discreditable to a University town' (p. 55). Ch. Four, 'Unemployment', helped remedy this, noting the undergraduates' ' "effective demands" ' for goods from the shops, and for services from their scouts and the unseen army dependent on their desires' (pp. 81–2).

60 C. H. Lee, 'Regional growth and structural change in the Victorian economy', *Economic History Review*, 2nd ser. XXXIV, 1981, p. 448.

61 Graham, 'The Suburbs', p. 18.

62 P. W. S. Andrews and E. Brunner, *The Eagle Ironworks, Oxford. The story of W. Lucy and Co. Ltd.*, Oxford, 1965; A. E. Coppard, *It's Me, O Lord!*, London, 1957; *Frank Cooper Ltd.*, brochure in Oxford City Library, Colchester, *c.* 1960.

63 'Death of the Late Mr Edward Radbone, 10 May 1905', in G. A. Oxon a. 22 f. 15; *The House of Grimbly, Hughes*, London, *c.* 1923.

64 See Butler, *Social Conditions, passim*.

65 Cf. *VCH*, p. 215.

66 University Archives, Minutes of Hebdomadal Council (26 November 1883).

67 PRO BT 31/14338/365c Clarendon Hotel Co. Ltd.

68 *DNB*; N. A. Rupke, *The Great Chain of History: William Buckland and the English School of Geology (1814–1844)*, Oxford, 1983, p. 13.

69 Bodl. G. A. Oxon. b 163 [City 15], misc. re. Oxford Electricity Co. 1892; PRO, BT 31/31257/34685. The company had some university links among directors and investors but over 95 per cent of the capital belonged to Sir Daniel Cooper, returned Sydney merchant and agent-general for New South Wales.

70 Ward, *Oxford*, 123; *VCH*, p. 211; J. Pycroft, *Oxford Memories*, 2 vols., London, 1886, pp. 34ff, chs. xii, xiii.

71 Bodl. Carlyle Mss, Eng. Lett. *c.* 481, E. L. Woodward to F. M. Powicke, 30 April [1944], recalling Carlyle's activities.

72 G. D. H. Cole and G. N. Clark, *The Tram Strike, a letter to City and University*, London, May 1913.

73 For a recent example, see A. Fox, *A Very Late Development*, Warwick, 1990.

74 R. J. Morris, 'Religion and medicine in 19th century Oxford', *Medical History*, London, 1975.

75 See, *inter alia*, W. Thorp and V. Thomas, *St Giles' Fair. Caution and Remonstrance. To all drunkards and revellers and to the thoughtless and imprudent of both sexes*, Oxford, 1 September 1832.

76 E.g. W. P. Ormerod, *On the Sanatory Condition of Oxford*, Oxford, Ashmolean Society, 1848.

77 Ormerod, *Sanatory Condition*, pp. 44 – 5.

78 It was, of course, during the vacation. See J. B. Atlay, *Sir Henry Wentworth Acland, Bart., K. C. B., F. R. S.: a memoir*, London, 1903, pp. 189 – 90.

79 Bodl. Acland Papers, d. 66.

80 PRO MH 13/141 Oxford Correspondence with General Board of Health and Local Government Office, 1848 – 71.

81 Liddell, Dean of Christ Church, was particularly sensitive to the dangers of disease, his period as Headmaster of Westminster having coincided with an outbreak of typhoid fever.

82 Partly they believed through absence, partly through the ill feeling in view of university opposition to the GWR works in that year. Acland Papers, Ms *d*. 69, *f*. 60 Liddell to Acland, 29 August 1865.

83 PRO MH 12/9716 Drainage scheme applications; Graham, p. 373.

84 Atlay, *Acland, passim*; *VCH*, p. 239.

85 E.g. *Provincial Hospitals*, London, 1875 *passim*; Oriel College, Oxford, Phelps Papers, Acland to Phelps, 11 June 1890.

86 Acland Ms *d*. 76 E. Alden, 16 November 1889, R. Buckell, 4 June 1890, G. C. Druce, n.d. (1890s) to Acland.

87 H. L. Thompson, *Henry George Liddell D. D.*, London, 1899, pp. 195 – 8.

88 *Politics*, 2 vols., 1885, ii, Preface; E. Abbott and L. Campbell, *The Life and Letters of Benjamin Jowett*, 2 vols., London, 1897, ii, pp. 219ff.

89 University Archives, Minutes of Hebdomadal Council, 13 February 1865; *Parliamentary Papers, 1865 XII (399)*, Thames River, evidence of Ald. W. Ward, q. 790; Thompson, *Henry Liddell, D. D.*, London, 1899, pp. 195ff.

90 E.g. J. Prestwich, *A Letter on the Oxford water supply*, Oxford, 1884.

91 University Archives, MR/3/3/2 Leaflet, *Thames Valley Drainage*, October 1883 with list of first subscribers.

92 University Archives, numerous ephemera, and leaflets of Faussett, e.g. *The Proposed Abolition of Iffley Lock*, 1885; MR/3/3/4 B. Price to Jowett, 23 October 1886.

93 *Oxford Valley Drainage. Retention of Iffley Lock*, leaflets, 15 June 1885, August 1886, in University Archives, MR 3/3/4.

94 *Oxford Water Supply. Letters and Report*, Oxford, 1885.

95 G. W. Child, *The Removal of Iffley Lock considered in relation to the Health of Oxford*, Oxford, 1885.

96 In effect, subscriptions were paid back, with a portion deducted to repay Jowett and Liddell for the expenses they had incurred. This work fell to Alfred Robinson, Bursar of New College, and Treasurer of the 'Abolitionists'. It was only completed after Jowett's death. MR/3/3/3 *passim*, e.g. Jowett to Robinson, 22 May 1889.

97 (World's Classics, Oxford, 1987); Mr Ward, don at Brasenose, was later a writer for *The Times*. See above, p. 18; Mrs H. Ward, *A Writer's Recollections*, 2 vols., London, 1918.

98 *Elsmere*, p. 76.

99 M. Richter, *The Politics of Conscience: T. H. Green and His Age*, London, 1964, esp. ch. 11; P. P. Nicholson, 'T. H. Green and state action: liquor legislation', *History of Political Thought*, London, VI, 1985, pp. 517–50.

100 Balliol College, Oxford, T. H. Green Papers, T. H. Green, Diary, 1874, *passim*.

101 For Colegrove, see M. B. Rix, *Life of Emma Mathews (née Colegrove)*, Oxford, 1960.

102 Green Papers, copy, C. A. Fyffe to *The Times*, 27 March 1882.

103 Green Papers, Mrs. C. M. Green, 'Notes on Green at Rugby, early Oxford days, and ideal of Christian citizenship'.

104 College servants, considered by some councillors as virtual members of the University, had held civic office, for example, Henry Grant, Sheriff in 1864. *Report of the Oxford Town Council Meeting, 9 Nov. 1864*, Oxford, 1864.

105 Toynbee failed to win the seat after Green's death. See Toynbee to B. R. Wise, Wise Papers, 23 Oct. 1882, Mitchell Library, Sydney; A. Kadish, *Apostle Arnold: The Life and Death of Arnold Toynbee*, Durham, NC, 1986, pp. 155–73.

106 R. L. Nettleship (ed.), *Works of Thomas Hill Green. Vol. 3 Miscellanies and Memoir*, London, 1888, 'Lecture on the Work to be done by the New Oxford High School for Boys', pp. 456–76.

107 New College, Oxford, W. A. Spooner, Draft Autobiography, 'Fifty Years in an Oxford College', p. 117; Brodrick, *Memories*, p. 386.

108 *Oxford Magazine*, 7 November 1929; Balliol College, Jowett Papers, C. M. Green to R. L. Nettleship, 24 December 1887, 'Time seems very long, though life has much that is beautiful and I am thankful to be well and able to go on alone – and do what my Husband wanted me to do – to make friends with working people and help them if I could that way.'

109 F. Haverfield (ed.), *H. Nettleship: Lectures and Essays*, Oxford, 1895, p. xxxiv; Bodl. G. A. Oxon b. 160 (93–6), Papers, East Oxford British School. Nor should one forget the earlier endeavours of Christian Socialists and Positivists, e.g. the Oxford Working Men's Educational Institution of 1856. See V. Morton, *Oxford Rebel: the life of N. S. Maskelyne*, Gloucester, 1986.

110 Thus, a Provost of Oriel in the 1920s, Phelps regularly took his young colleagues to visit the Cowley Road workhouse; conversation with the late Eric Hargreaves, Oriel College, *c*. 1977.

111 Phelps, *Poor Law and Charity*, Oxford, 1887; 'Rules for the Guidance of Guardians in their Administration of Relief' and 'Statement of the Rev. L. R. Phelps, MA, 30 Apr. 1888', in Bodl. G. A. Oxon b. 165; *The Administration of the Poor Law in Oxford*, Oxford, 1900.

112   Beatrice Webb recorded Phelps as contemplating signing both Majority and Minority Reports in 1907. *The Diary of Beatrice Webb, vol. 3 1905–1914*, London, 1984, p. 88.

113   Phelps Papers, Hall to Phelps, 26 June, 11 and 27 July 1887; *VCH*, p. 349.

114   J. T. Dodd, *A Lecture on "Poor Law Administration with particular reference to Out-relief in Oxford"*, Oxford, 1899.

115   For the conflict between these groups, which led to the election of the 'weak' G. W. Cooper as chairman in 1902 rather than Phelps, see J. C. Wilson to Phelps, Phelps Papers, 25 and 28 March 1902.

116   T. H. Kingerlee, *Letter to Heads and Bursars of Colleges who elect Guardians to the Oxford Union*, Oxford, 1900; cf. dons, H. W. B. Joseph, *The Administration of Poor Relief in the Oxford Incorporation*, Oxford, 1900, and J. C. Wilson, *Poor Law Administration in Oxford*, 26 February 1900. For Wilson, one of the founders of Jurisprudence at Oxford, see *Oxford Magazine*, 15 February 1905. Kingerlee and his colleagues were also later largely responsible for organising relief works under the Oxford Unemployed Relief Committee; see Report, 1911–12 in Bodl. G. A. Oxon b. 162(54); British Library of Political and Economic Science, Webb Local Government Collection, vol. 333 for the origins of this committee in 1907.

117   W. S. Holdsworth, W. H. Hughes, and W. M. Merry, *Poor Law Representation within the Oxford Incorporation*, Oxford, 1902; Wilson considered the authors 'old ignoramuses'. To Phelps, 28 March 1902. See also J. G. Talbot (University MP) to Phelps, 2 and 14 April 1903.

118   Cf. B. Harrison, 'Miss Butler's Oxford Survey', in A. H. Halsey (ed.), *Traditions of Social Policy*, Oxford, 1975, pp. 27–72, where local divisions over Poor Law policy are ignored.

119   Oxford COS, *Annual Report, 1913*, p. 9.

120   Butler, *Oxford*, p. 252.

121   See above, p. 14.

122   Coppard, *It's me*, p. 155.

123   Halsey (ed.), *Social Policy, passim*.

124   This is not of course a complete view, even of Edwardian Oxford. It omits influential dons like A. J. Carlyle. See Harrison's account of Oxford's 'reforming elite' in Halsey, *Social Policy* and also Whiting, *Cowley*, ch. 1.

125   *Oxford Chronicle*, 15 November 1907.

126   Oman, *Victorian Oxford*, pp. 177–8, citing Plumptre.

127   All plays in term-time required his sanction. Dons, notably 'Lewis Carroll' (C. H. Dodgson), often urged the exercise of this power in the interests of morality and discipline.

128   E.g. S. F. Hulton, *Rixae Oxoniensis*, Oxford, 1892.

129   *VCH*, pp. 234–6.

130   PRO MH 12/9706 T. Mallam, jun. to Poor Law Commission, 18 November 1842.

131 F.J. Morrell, *Oxford Paving Bill* (3 April 1848).

132 'Town and gown in 1848', *Oxford Protestant Magazine*, May 1848, pp. 44–8; G. Eyre, *To the Ratepayers ... in the City of Oxford, Oxford, 1852.*

133 L. L. Shadwell, *Enactments in Parliament specially concerning the Universities of Oxford and Cambridge*, Oxford Historical Society, 4 vols., Oxford 1912, iii, pp. 173–85.

134 Kadish, *Apostle Arnold*, p. 169; for a review of this issue, see C. Neate, *The Answer of Charles Neate to a Recent Vote of Convocation*, Oxford, ?1857.

135 C. Neate, *On the Proper Share of the University in the Board of Street Commissioners*, Oxford, 1854.

136 *VCH*, p. 233.

137 PRO MH12/141 C.J. Sadler (Mayor) to Sir B. Hall, 30 December 1854.

138 Shadwell, *Enactments*, iii, pp. 289–91.

139 Neate, *Proper Share, passim.*

140 Bodl. Ms Top Oxon b. 172 Local Government Papers, Oxford Paving Acts (f14); Ms Top Oxon e. 292 St Clements' Turnpike and Oxford Paving Acts. Rough Minutes. 1858–60.

141 PRO MH13/141 Oxford Correspondence, 1855–66.

142 Oxfordshire Record Office, R5 Oxford Local Board, minutes. Taking 1876 as a random sample year, University members of the board attended an average of 6.1 meetings, townsmen, 11.3.

143 Shadwell, *Enactments*, iii, pp. 409–20; *VCH*, p. 230; Engel, 'Prostitution', pp. 99–100. Both the prospect of the railway workshops in 1865 and the bread riots of 1867 had brought to the forefront the need for a solution to the police problem.

144 *VCH*, p. 240; C. Fenby, *The Other Oxford. The Life and Times of Frank Gray and his Father*, London, 1970.

145 PRO MH12/9721 J.J. Bickerton to Local Government Office, 4 July 1888.

146 PRO MH12/9721 Sir Hugh Owen, minute, 6 July, 1888.

147 University Archives, Hebdomadal Council Papers, 1887–88. A Committee on municipal administration was set up in January 1887. A Boundaries Committee followed.

148 PRO MH12/9721 Local Government Office, correspondence, 1888; *Jackson's Oxford Journal*, 3 November 1888.

149 J.C. Wilson, *The Proposed Agreement between the University and the City respecting the Local Government of Oxford*, 6 June and 12 December 1888.

150 PRO MH12/9721 Wilson to J.J. Henley, 22 September, 6 December 1888.

151 University Archives, Hebdomadal Council Papers, 30 April, 4, 9, and 18 June, 15, 20, 22, and 29 October, 5 and 11 November 1888; Shadwell, *Enactments*, iv, pp. 152–72.

152   Bodl. G.A. Oxon b. 162(26). Attendance at Council, 1897–98.

153   'useful experience of strange places', as Cannan wrote to Phelps, when lobbying for 'Progressive' University men on the Council. Phelps Papers, 23 September 1905.

154   Columbia University, New York, Seligman Papers, Cannan to Seligman, 22 January 1897; cf. Seligman to Cannan, 4 January 1897, Cannan Papers, BLPES. See too for Cannan's later reflections on local government, *The History of Local Rates*, London, 1912, pp. x – xi.

155   C.R.L. Fletcher (ed.), *Reliquae A.D. Godley*, 2 vols., Oxford, 1926, i, p. 3; *Oxford Magazine*, 15 October 1925, p. 69; *Oxford Magazine*, 17 May 1945. Few of Bowman's Merton colleagues could understand how he contrived to spend his time.

156   For example, Revd. H.J. George, whose chief interest remained 'the affairs of life'. *Oxford Magazine*, 27 April 1939.

157   Brodrick, *Memories*, pp. 382ff.

158   Bodl. G.A. Oxon a 22(20), 'The Late Alderman Saunders, JP' (1911).

159   Bodl. Tramways Papers, G.A. Oxon b. 162(70), 'The Tramways Question', Oxford Trades and Labour Council (1897).

160   Bodl. Tramways Papers, G.A. Oxon b. 162(70), Oxford Tramways, public meetings, 1902, 1905; 'The Proposed Purchase of the Tramway' (1905).

161   G.E. Baker *et al.*, *The the Ratepayers of Oxford. The Oxford Corporation Tram Bill* (22 January 1906); E. Cannan, *To the Resident Members of Congregation* (26 January 1906); A.J. Carlyle, 'The Tramways Question', *Oxford Magazine*, 1905, p. 393.

162   Bodl. G.A. Oxon b. 162(73) anti-tramways handbill, 1906. For Morris's role, see also Bodl. G.A. Oxon b. 162(90), 'A Right Merrye Tale', and P.W.S. Andrews and E. Brunner, *The Life of Lord Nuffield*, Oxford, 1955, pp. 20 – 3. See also Councillor Godley's celebrated verse, 'the Motor Bus' ('Yes, the smell and hideous hum / Indicat Motorem Bum'), 1914.

163   *Oxford Chronicle*, 12 January 1906; 2 February 1906. For 1117: Against 5092.

164   Above, p. 22; 'The Oxford Tram Strike', leaflet, 26 March 1913.

165   Supplement to *Oxford Chronicle*, 7 July 1863. Neate was unseated in 1857 but held the seat from 1863 to 1868.

166   Harvie, *Liberalism, passim.*

167   *Parliamentary Papers, 1857 Sess. 2 VIII(170)*, S.C. Oxford City Election Petition; *Parliamentary Papers, 1881, XLIV[C2856, 2856 –1]*, R.C. Oxford election, 1880.

168   For Sidgwick, see *Oxford Magazine*, 29 October 1920; F. Sidgwick (son) to T.H. Kingerlee, 27 July 1912 enclosed in Kingerlee's copy of C.V. Butler, *Social Conditions in Oxford* (copy in Oriel College Library).

169 Bodl. Oxford Liberal Association, annual reports, 1887 – 1915; Oxford Election Papers, 1892 – 1910; Phelps Papers, A. Sidgwick to Phelps, 1 January 1907.

170 S. M. Burrows (ed.), *Autobiography of Montagu Burrows*, London, 1908, pp. 231 – 6.

171 Oman, *Victorian Oxford*, pp. 145 – 6. Oman acquired an 'acute distaste for electioneering work'; Bodl. G. A. Oxon 40 274 Oxford Political Papers, for Poole and the Conservative Registration Association in 1892.

172 *VCH*, p. 254; Bodl. Misc. papers of Oxford Conservative, Liberal Unionist, and Women's Liberal Unionist Associations, 1889 – 1905.

173 *Parl. Papers, 1880, Sess-2, LVIII(349)*, Oxford Election petition; *1881, XLIV, [2856, 2856-I]*, Royal Commission, Oxford Election. In 1880, Magdalen Tower was reported as 'blue from top to bottom'; Eng. Lett d. 81, T. H. Green to A. Acland, 29 March 1880, for Faussett's attempt to eject a Liberal from his Christ Church tenement.

174 D. A. Talboys, *To the University of Oxford and Public in General*, November 1837). In 1835 and 1841 college servants provided a solid Tory block vote. J. Vincent, *Pollbooks: How the Victorians Voted*, Cambridge, 1963, pp. 158 – 9.

175 Oxford City Library, misc. papers of The Free Trade League of the University, City and County of Oxford, including *Report of A. W. Hall at Charlbury, 3 Jan. 1906*; Phelps Papers, Hall to Phelps, 24 December 1903; G. E. Underhill to Phelps, 2 October 19 and 21 November 1903.

176 Whiting, *Cowley, passim*.

177 As Chesney noted in the 1892 election, co-operation between classes provided a surer basis for modern civilisation than new public laws. Manifesto, June 1892 in Oxford Election Papers, Bodl.

178 Beerbohm, *Zuleika Dobson*, pp. 137 – 8.

179 Earl of Darnley (ed.), *Frank Lascelles, 'Our Modern Orpheus'*, Oxford, 1932, p. 92. See too 'Patriotism and pageantry', *Isis*, 22 June 1907, p. 418; Oman, *Victorian Oxford*, pp. 255 – 6; Carola Oman, *An Oxford Childhood*, London, 1976, pp. 96, 100 – 1.

180 *Oxford Times*, 6 July 1907, p. 7.

181 Not all were enthusiastic. T. B. Strong, Dean of Christ Church, had 'hoped that the boredom of the Pageant had cured us of bothering ourselves about our history, at any rate during the life of the present inhabitants of Oxford: but the prospect of anything else like this makes me wish that I lived at Port Sunlight or Tooting or Chicago'. Strong to F. Madan, 19 July 1911 in Madan's collection of Oxford Millenary Papers, Bodl.

182 A point spelt out by the progressive councillor for North Oxford, Basil Blackwell. *Oxford Chronicle*, 26 January 1912, p. 8.

183 *Oxford Chronicle*, 12 July 1912, *passim*; Butler's *Social Conditions* appearing in 1912 suitably noted 'the sense of common responsibility for the city' as a social bond, 'probably stronger now than in any of the previous centuries' (p. 246).

184   E.g. Brodrick, *Memories*, p. 346; Oman, *Victorian Oxford*, pp. 137 – 41; J. E. Courtney, *An Oxford Portrait Gallery*, London, 1931, pp. 209ff.

185   Ward, *Victorian Oxford*, p. 301.

186   Oman, *Victorian Oxford*, 259.

187   The old order is well depicted in M. J. Gifford, *Pages from the Diary of an Oxford Lady, 1843–1862*, Oxford, 1932; the new in Harrison, 'Miss Butler', and C. Colvin, 'A don's wife a century ago', *Oxoniensa*, L, 1985, pp. 267–78; *Oxford Magazine*, XI, 1892–93, p. 313, obituary of Margaret Evans. See also Peretz, below, *passim*.

188   For adverse reactions to the social and political impact of women in Oxford, see Brodrick, p. 387 and B. Brown (ed.), *The England of Henry Taunt: Victorian Photographer*, London, 1973, p. 170.

Architecture and townscape since 1800

In the 1830s, according to the Revd W. Tuckwell,

the approach to Oxford by the Henley road was the most beautiful in the world. Soon after passing Littlemore you came in sight of, and did not lose again, the sweet city with its dreaming spires, driven along a road crowded and obscured with dwellings, open then to cornfields on the right, to uninclosed meadows on the left, with an unbroken view of the long line of towers, rising out of foliage less high and veiling than after sixty more years of growth today. At once, without suburban interval, you entered the finest quarter of the town, rolling under Magdalen Tower and past the Magdalen elms, then in full unmutilated luxuriance, till the exquisite curves of the High Street opened on you.[1]

At that time, 'railroads and enclosures had not girdled Oxford proper wtih a coarse suburban fringe. On the three approaches to the town, the Henley, Banbury, Abingdon roads, it was cut off, clear as a walled and gated Jericho, from adjacent country.'[2] This was the city whose magic so enchanted the sensitive soul of the undergraduate John Henry Newman.

'City' was, of course, its appellation by right, since the see of Oxford had been established by Henry VIII, and it was a county town too, but its appearance must have been that of a market town of moderate size, whose architectural distinction was due entirely to the University. Even the Cathedral formed part of a college, and though there were fourteen parish churches of medieval foundation, the only ones of substantial size and presence were those of St Mary Virgin, which doubled as the University Church, and St John the Baptist, which also served as the chapel of Merton College. There was the modest Town Hall, by Isaac Ware, dating from 1751–52, but Otho Nicholson's splendid great Conduit of 1616 had been removed from the nearby Carfax to the park of Nuneham Courtenay in 1787. In the High Street were John Gwynn's handsome Markets of 1773–74, and, as Surveyor to the Oxford Paving Commissioners, he was also architect for the dignified Magdalen Bridge (1772–90) at its other end, and for the Workhouse (1772–75), on the site where Wellington Square now is. There were the two gaols, the county one, in the castle (begun by William Blackburn in around 1785 and completed in 1805 by Daniel Harris), and the city one on Gloucester Green (1786–89, also by Blackburn). The Radcliffe Infirmary (1759–70, by Stiff Leadbetter) was a benefaction from the Trustees of Dr Radcliffe, who mostly benefited the University, as was the Radcliffe Observatory, also to the north-west of the town centre (1772–94, by Henry Keene and James Wyatt).

None of these buildings could begin to match the great show-pieces of the University. The medieval glories of the finest colleges (Merton, New College, Magdalen, All Souls, Christ Church) had almost been outshone by the magnificent constructions of the eighteenth century, which put Oxford in the forefront of architectural taste. These included the Clarendon Building, the North Quadrangle of All Souls, Queen's College, Christ Church Library, and the Radcliffe Camera. However, the architectural character of the University as a whole was predominantly of the seventeenth century, and mostly old-fashioned for its date, though there were outstanding exceptions in the Canterbury Quadrangle at St John's, the Botanic Garden gateway, the old Ashmolean Museum, and the Sheldonian Theatre. The general character of the city's domestic architecture, as can still be seen, for example, on the north side of Holywell Street, and as can be poignantly experienced in the water-colours of J. C. Buckler,[3] was mostly in an attractive but undistinguished vernacular, with only an occasional exception such as 'Vanbrugh House' in St Michael's Street, or the equally Vanbrughian house that stood at the corner of Catte Street and Holywell, showing the influence of the great architects who worked for the University. Many of the houses were dressed up around the turn of the century in stucco, with bay windows and straight roof lines.[4] The University had less effect on the town than might have been expected, for its members lived a monastic life in their colleges, only the most senior being allowed to marry, so that they did not require accommodation elsewhere in town. Nor were their commercial needs likely to affect the character of the town, except on a limited scale.

By the beginning of the nineteenth century, some junior members of the University must have been living out, for in 1809 a statute was passed 'prohibiting more strictly than ever residence out of College'.[5] This led to a certain amount of building by a few colleges, but the only major project of the first quarter of the century was the new Magdalen Hall, in Catte Street, by William Garbett (1820–22), built by Magdalen College to free the land previously occupied by the Hall for its own expansion. Magdalen Hall (now Hertford College) was classical in style, but by this date many felt that this was wrong for Oxford. It was already fashionable to replace parapets with battlements (despite the fact that Loggan's seventeenth-century views show that these were rare), and to add Gothic details to earlier buildings.

A good deal of this work was done by Daniel Robertson, who came to Oxford as an architect for the first major building erected in the nineteenth century by the University. This was to house its Press, for the flourishing demand for bibles and prayer-books meant that its premises in the Clarendon Building were much too cramped. The new building, erected between 1825 and 1829, was sited well away from the town centre, on what is now Walton Street: this was presumably because it was intended from the first to use steam power (though the first engine was not installed until 1834). The site no doubt also explains why Robertson felt free to use the classical style, providing an amazingly grand triumphal arch entrance with Corinthian columns. The siting of the Press may also have been due to the proximity of the Oxford Canal, opened in 1790, as was that of Lucy's Eagle Ironworks, established in 1825 a little further north. The result was that this part of Oxford took on a working-class character, and in 1836 it acquired a church, designed by Henry Jones Underwood in the Greek Revival style. Underwood had come to Oxford in 1830 to supervise Sir Robert Smirke's alterations to the Bodleian Library, and he succeeded Robertson, who had made a precipitate departure from Oxford in 1829, as the principal local architect.

Two other new churches had already been built in growing suburbs. St Clement's, replacing an old predecessor on a new site, was built between 1825 and 1828 by Robertson in a Norman style so cack-handed that it became known as 'The Roasted Hare', while for the expanding village of Summertown the more seemly church of St John was designed by Underwood. Present at its consecration in 1833 was the vicar of the Church of St Mary the Virgin, J.H. Newman. The early English style of St John's was taken from its mother-church of St Giles, and Newman used both the architect and the style for the church which he built in the village of Littlemore which, though two miles out of Oxford, formed part of his parish. This simple but dignified building, consecrated in 1836, was much admired and imitated.[6] In 1845 *The Ecclesiologist* described it as 'the first unqualified step to better things that England had long witnessed'.[7] *The Ecclesiologist* was the journal of the Cambridge Camden (later Ecclesiological) Society. This was founded in May 1839, but had been preceded, by a few months, by the Oxford Society for Promoting the Study of Gothic Architecture (OSPSGA). This body, 'from the beginning a highly respectable society supported by the academic élite of Oxford' was, although less widely known than its Cambridge counterpart, to exert a great influence on architecture, through lectures, collections of casts and the like, and publications.[8] These latter included in 1840 *Elevations, Sections and Details of the Church of St Mary the Virgin at Littlemore, Oxfordshire.*

The association with Newman draws attention to the obvious fact that this new serious approach to Gothic architecture was closely associated with the Catholic revival in the Church of England, known as the Oxford Movement, and usually dated from the Assize Sermon preached by John Keble in 1833. The Protestant backlash, however, saw no need to repudiate authentic Gothic: nothing could have shown this more clearly than its physical expression in the form of the Martyrs' Memorial, erected immediately north of the Church of St Mary Magdalen (to which an aisle was added as part of the project) between 1841 and 1843. Commemorating Cranmer, Latimer, and Ridley, who had been burnt under Mary, it was a result of a competition, which stipulated that the design should be based on the Eleanor Cross at Waltham. The winner was the young George Gilbert Scott.

A year earlier, another competition had been held for a more important structure, on a site close by, at the corner of the newly-constructed Beaumont Street.[9] The University had decided to put up a building to house two separate institutions, one for the study of modern languages, in accordance with the will of Sir Robert Taylor, the other to house its collection of ancient marbles and other works of art. Designs had to be 'of Grecian character' to suit the antiquities, and the winner was Charles Robert Cockerell, the

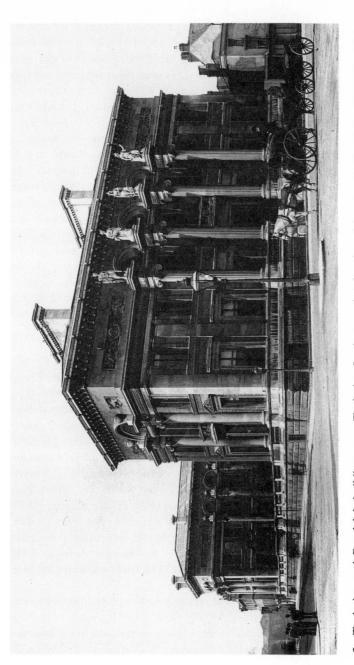

2 Taylorian and Randolph building, now Taylorian Institute and Ashmolean Museum (C.R. Cockerell, 1841–45), from St Giles. *Oxfordshire Photographic Archive*

most learned and also the most inventive classical architect in England. He was given a remarkably free hand, and the building which went up between 1841 and 1845 was an astonishing synthesis of elements not only from Greece and Rome, but also from sixteenth-century Italy and eighteenth-century England. It was enormously expensive, costing almost £50,000: apart from Taylor's bequest, a large sum came from profits of the University Press.

Not everyone liked the new building. In his *Apology for the Revival of Christian Architecture in England* (1843), A.W.N. Pugin raged: 'the man who paganises *in the Universities* deserves no quarter'. In the same year came Pugin's own great opportunity at Oxford, when he was asked to produce designs for the rebuilding of most of the main quadrangle of Balliol College. Basically medieval, this had been partly rebuilt between 1738 and 1743, but its stonework was fearfully decayed. Pugin's designs were entrancing, but the architect he superseded, George Basevi, was outraged, and a 'civil war' broke out among the Fellows, largely on religious grounds.[10] As a result, Pugin's scheme was shelved, and his only works at Oxford were a gateway for Magdalen, erected in 1844, but removed in 1883, and two stained-glass windows (made by Wailes) in St Mary the Virgin, to two children of the actor George Bartley.

In the 1840s almost everything built for the University was Gothic. University College went to Sir Charles Barry, architect of the Palace of Westminster, for a new block of rooms on High Street (1840–42), while Pembroke, for extensive new buildings which included a grandiose hall, chose John Hayward, from Exeter. Magdalen looked nearer home for an architect for its Choristers' School Hall (now the Library), designed by John Chessell Buckler, son of the College's London bailiff. In the same decade three new churches went up, all Gothic. In the centre was St George's, in George Street, by James Park Harrison (1849–50). Underwood built Holy Trinity Church (1845) to serve the southern part of St Ebbe's parish. The third church, also dedicated to the Trinity, catered for the increasing population of the village of Headington Quarry: it was built between 1848 and 1849 to the design of G.G. Scott. The first two have now been demolished.

For their new County Hall, erected in New Road between 1839 and 1841, the magistrates chose not Gothic, but Norman, because of the proximity of the Castle. Their architect was the local John Plowman. He had rebuilt St Martin's Church, at Carfax, in a thoroughly incorrect Gothic between 1820 and 1822, but, no doubt as a result of the influence both of his sadly short-lived but far more talented son, Thomas (*c.* 1805 – 28), and of the OSPSGA, had somewhat mended his ways. All the same, he used the classical style for one ecclesiastical structure, though a far from conventional one – the Floating Chapel, built for the canal boatmen in 1839 (unfortunately it sank in around 1868). The magistrates again chose Norman, for the same reason, for the County Police Station, also in New Road, designed by Buckler.

The Gothic (or Tudor style) was surprisingly slow in affecting domestic architecture in and around Oxford. For the detached villas built in the suburbs in these decades, the classical style was generally preferred, with only the odd exception such as Gothic Cottage in Summertown (1831), or The Priory at Iffley. Particularly striking was the Italianate style of Park Town, built between 1853 and 1855 by Samuel Lipscomb Seckham, a local man who had learned his business in London.[11]

For college works, a rather old-fashioned late Gothic style could still be used in the 1850s, as for example by the country house architect Anthony Salvin at Balliol (1852 – 53), and by J. C. Buckler: in partnership with his son Charles Alban, he gave Jesus College the pleasant front which represents most people's idea of the typical Oxford College (1854 – 56). But these were the years when several much bolder works were to bring Oxford into the limelight. The first of these was the new chapel designed for Balliol by William Butterfield in 1854. Its most remarkable features were not its geometrical decorated Gothic, nor its steeply-pitched roof and idiosyncratic bell-turret, but its materials and detailing – the exterior of alternate courses of red and yellow stone, the richly coloured interior lined with inlaid alabaster and fitted out in Butterfield's very personal manner.

Balliol Chapel did not meet with the approval it deserved. Far more acceptable was the new chapel erected on the other side of Broad Street, in 1856 – 59, by G. G. Scott. Its unsatisfactory siting was due to vacillations only too typical of college governing bodies, but the building itself was a powerful demonstration of the way foreign influences were affecting English architecture. Its lofty proportions, its apse, and its stone vaulting were of the obviously French derivation (though its similarity to the Sainte-Chapelle is less close than is often maintained). The rich decoration – stone-carving, wood-carving, brass and ironwork, encaustic tiles, inlaid marble, mosaics, and stained glass – was typical of the elaborately harmonious setting now desired for Anglican collegiate worship.

Splendid as these chapels were, they were of a conventional building type, but the other major work of the 1850s was not. This was the University Museum, whose importance and influence, both inside and outside Oxford, can hardly be overemphasised. Its origins and concept were as revolutionary as its architecture. The provision for both the teaching of science and the housing of scientific collections in Oxford was appalling. A group of doughty fighters, led by Dr Henry Acland, was determined to remedy this, and in 1849 secured a resolution to the effect that a museum should be built to assemble all the materials explanatory of the earth and of the organic beings placed upon it, together with teaching accommodation. The scheme was at last accepted by Convocation in 1853, and a site in the Parks was bought. A competition was held, laying down that the area with three sides of a quadrangle should be 'covered in by a glass roof', and that the Chemical Laboratory and Dissecting Rooms should be detached, for obvious reasons. The cost could not exceed £30,000. Once again, the money came from the profits of the Press. Eventually Convocation was faced with a choice between a Renaissance design by Edward Middleton Barry (son of Sir Charles), and a 'Rhenish Gothic' one by the Irish firm of Deane and Woodward.

It was hardly surprising that the latter won. The responsibility for it really belonged to the scholarly Benjamin Woodward, a silent man possessed of extraordinary personal magnetism. Work began in 1855, and the Museum opened in 1860. Woodward's design, with its sheer façade symmetrically arranged about a central tower, was quite novel for a public building. Its style owed a great deal to North Italy, and the influence of Ruskin was crucial, though his direct role in the conception and execution of the building was less extensive than has often been claimed. The elaborate stone-carving, both inside and out, relates to the Museum's teaching programme, showing botanical and (rather peculiar) zoological specimens, while the shafts of the arcading on the two storeys around the quadrangle were of polished stones from around Britain. The carving was done by the wild Irish team of John and James O'Shea and Edward Whelan. The iron and glass roof of the quadrangle (intended as the museum proper) was undertaken by Francis Skidmore of Coventry, known for ecclesiastical metalwork: it caused tremendous problems, especially because Skidmore decided to use wrought iron

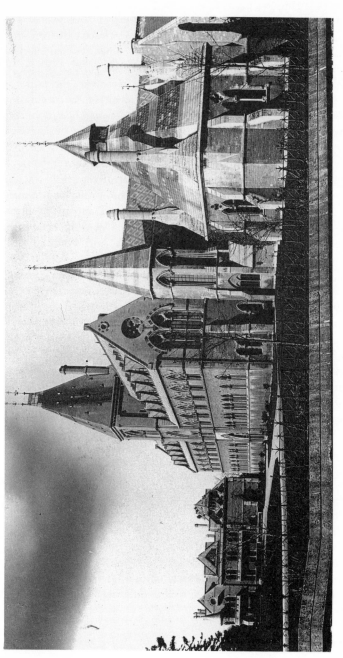

3 University Museum (Deane and Woodward, 1855–60), and former Clarendon (Physics) Laboratory (T. N. Deane, 1867–69). *Oxfordshire Photographic Archive*

for the shafts, instead of the cast iron specified by Woodward. The roof started to fail, and Skidmore had to substitute cast iron after all. The interior was further elaborated with Woodward's characteristic notched and pierced woodwork, statues of distinguished scientists, and painted decoration in teaching rooms. However, the museum was constantly starved of funds, so that much of the decoration was left unexecuted.

The building of the Museum aroused extraordinary excitement in Oxford, since it seemed to be reconciling science and art in a new way. Architecturally, it had the effect of securing the triumph of Gothic for at least twenty years. The most direct result was the number of commissions given to Woodward and (after his untimely death in 1861 at the age of forty-four) to his partner Thomas Newenham Deane. The most important was the Union Debating Hall (now Library) of 1856. Here Woodward used brick, and the steep roof, and sheer walls with windows set back within them, clearly show Ruskin's influence. The interior is famous for the wall-paintings unsuccessfully executed by Dante Gabriel Rossetti and his young friends: these included William Morris and Edward Burne-Jones, who had met as undergraduates at Exeter College (1853 – 55). Woodward's other works included a new east window for the Latin Chapel of Christ Church Cathedral, which was filled with jewel-like glass designed by Burne-Jones and made by Powell's, and additions to two private houses (one of them Acland's).

The uncompromising Gothic of these works set the fashion for the new suburb of North Oxford that was at last beginning to get under way,[12] and it was in this suburb that, in the year the Museum was opened, work began on another building which was to be of national importance. This was the church intended to cater for its residents. Dedicated to SS Philip and James, it was designed by George Edmund Street, one of the greatest of all nineteenth-century architects. He had close connections with Oxford, for he had an office in the city from 1852 to 1856, and he was Diocesan Architect from 1850 until his death in 1881, but it is surprising how little work he did in the town. His only executed work for the University was the restoration of Jesus College Chapel, but he did a fair amount of work in the parish churches, as well as building St Ebbe's Rectory and schools for St Ebbe's and St Paul's. However, SS Philip and James is one of his best churches. 'This noble building', according to Paul Joyce, 'occupies a crucial position in the progress of High

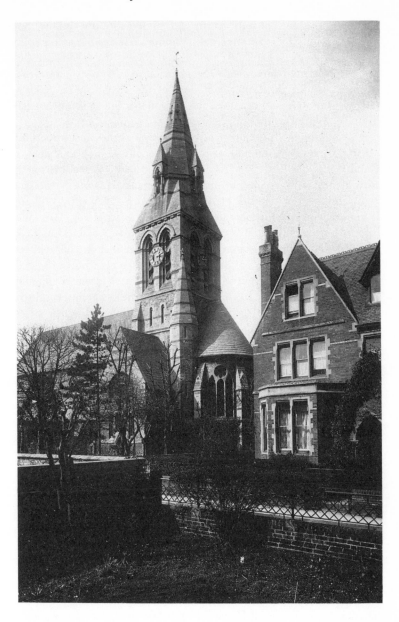

4   Church of SS Philip and James (G. E. Street, 1860–65) with no. 1 Church Walk (Frederick Codd, 1876). *Oxfordshire Photographic Archive*

Victorian Gothic, not only for its radical stylistic innovations, but also by reason of its experimental planning'.[13] It has a massive spire over the crossing, an apsidal chancel, and a nave whose wide arcades are boldly canted in towards the chancel arch. It was excessively strong meat for the tamer members of the Architectural Society (as the OSPSGA had renamed itself in 1848), but it could not fail to make an impression.

By the mid-1860s Oxford had become one of the most important centres of modern architecture in the country, far outstripping Cambridge. The bravery of its academic patrons was demonstrated, with breathtaking results, in the glorious transformation of the late eighteenth-century interior of Worcester College Chapel by William Burges. Using all his unmatched resources of learning, art, and colour, he not only fitted it out for contemporary worship but gave it richly symbolic iconography. Another intelligent choice of architect was made by the Fellows of Balliol in 1866, when at last they decided to replace the main front of the College. The Master, Benjamin Jowett, explained that, in choosing the Manchester architect Alfred Waterhouse, 'we hope to avoid eccentricity and un-English styles and fancies. Simplicity and proportion and not colour always seemed to me to be the great merits of architecture'.[14] This shows how much Jowett disliked Butterfield's Chapel, but what he got from Waterhouse was anything but the feebly traditional design his words might suggest: its heroic proportions, practical sash-windows, and vigorous detailings are very much of their time. Waterhouse is at last recognised as one of the artistic giants of Victorian architecture: he did even more work at Cambridge, but at Oxford he was employed again for the new hall and flanking buildings at Balliol (1873–77), and the new debating hall for the Union Society (1878), where, in an out-of-the-way situation, he used the teracotta of which he was so fond.

In North Oxford the favoured style of the principal architects – William Wilkinson, Charles Buckeridge, and Frederick Codd – was a vigorous and manly High Victorian Gothic, in yellow or red brick, with picturesque but unfussy proportions, and a good deal of elaborate stone-carving. The latter was readily available in the city, because of the number of the masons working there, on the constant repairs needed by buildings not only old, but comparatively new, but built in the poor Headington stone. For example, it is not always realised just how completely Queen's College was renewed.

It was on the edge of the new suburb, and immediately opposite the new Museum, that another building of the highest importance arose. This was the first college founded *de novo* since the Reformation. Its origins are of great interest in themselves. Since the 1840s there had been a growing demand for what was called 'University extension' – the widening of the possibility of university education. The cause was particularly espoused by the High Church party, for the universities were the most common route into the Anglican priesthood. However, they were also alarmed at the growing secularisation of the University, with the abolition of the religious tests which had kept out dissenters. The obvious course was to found a new college, and the death of John Keble in 1866 provided the opportunity. The new College, to be named in his memory, would (according to its charter) be one 'wherein sober living and high culture of the mind may be combined with Christian training based upon the principles of the Church of England'. These ideals were embodied in the architecture, and no more suitable architect could have been found than William Butterfield. A committed High Churchman himself, and well known to the founders of Keble through his High Church associations, he was noted for his radical approach to planning and design. The buildings were begun in 1868, and were complete, in all essentials, by 1883. This was made possible by generous benefactors.

The planning of the College was daringly unconventional. The great main quadrangle is appropriately dominated by the massive chapel, opposite which the hall and library are at first-floor level, over the common rooms. Butterfield regularised the declivities left by the gravel-digging to provide a terraced effect to the quadrangle which exaggerates the height of the buildings. A striking innovation was that the rooms were reached not off staircases, as was traditional in Oxford, but off corridors. This was primarily for economic reasons, as such residential blocks were reckoned to be cheaper both to build and to service. A smaller and less regular southern quadrangle included the bursary, lecture room, and 'Servants' Building', while at the south-east corner was the Warden's Lodging. The interior of the vaulted chapel was gorgeously decorated with inlaid marble and alabaster, mosaics, and stained glass, to a powerful iconographical scheme devised by Butterfield himself. The hall was the longest in Oxford, not from bravado, but to seat the whole College at once – another economy.

However, the most obviously striking, and controversial feature of Keble was its building material – brick, and polychrome brick at that, laid in elaborate patterns. Butterfield quite reasonably defended his choice on a number of grounds: not only was brick cheaper, but it resisted fire better, it was the material for the neighbouring suburban houses, and polychrome patterned brick was a local tradition in South Oxfordshire and Berkshire. He himself described the walls as 'gay'.

The 1860s and 1870s saw the triumph of High Victorian Gothic in the town too, in all types of architecture. An exception, however, was the most unusual church built to serve the suburb of Jericho: as this was largely inhabited by employees of the University Press, the Church of St Barnabas was the gift of Thomas Combe, Superintendent of the Press. Best known today as a patron of the Pre-Raphaelites, he was a staunch High Churchman, and had already built a Gothic chapel (consecrated in 1865) for the Radcliffe Infirmary. Its architect was Arthur Blomfield, son of the bishop of London, and well known for church work. He was chosen again for St Barnabas, where Combe demanded solidity without extravagance: the result, built between 1868 and 1869, was in the style of an Italian Romanesque basilica, well suited for Tractarian ritual. It was built of rendered rubble with brick bands, but much cast concrete was also used. A tall campanile was added in 1872. Thomas Hardy (who had worked for Blomfield) represents the church as St Silas in *Jude the Obscure*.

Another eminent church architect, S. S. Teulon, designed St Frideswide's, to serve Osney Town, in a chunky Gothic (1870–72): it never received its intended spire. The Jesuits employed the veteran Roman Catholic architect, Joseph Aloysius Hansom (assisted by his son Joseph Stanislas), for their Gothic church of St Aloysius in Woodstock Road. Its single apsidal vessel, with narrow 'passage-aisles', was very up-to-date (1873–75). Even the Methodists built a church with a tall spire, the Wesley Memorial in New Inn Hall Street (1878), though its architect, Charles Bell, was no great artist. The new church completely upstaged its plain classical predecessor of 1817–18, which was characteristic of the Nonconformist places of worship of the early nineteenth century, of which a surviving example is the Baptist Church in New Road (1819, by John Hudson).

The growing suburb of Cowley acquired a new parish church, dedicated to SS Mary and John, and built in stages between 1875 and 1893: its unadventurous Gothic was due to a local man, Alfred Mardon Mowbray. More interesting architecturally was St John's

Hospital for Incurables, of which the first part was begun just behind the site of the new church, in 1873. It was run by Anglican nuns. Its architect was another local man, Charles Buckeridge, an able Goth who died in the same year aged only forty.[15] He had designed other good buildings in the town, including the Probate Registry in New Road (1863), two houses in Norham Gardens, the Savings Bank (now demolished) in St Aldate's (1867–68), and the first purpose-built religious house. This was Holy Trinity Convent, near SS Philip and James in Woodstock Road. Buckeridge's amazing first design had a plan based on the medieval symbol of the Trinity, but what was built between 1866 and 1868, in a severe but handsome Gothic, was more conventional. The lofty apsed chapel was not built until 1891–94, but J. L. Pearson followed Buckeridge's design closely.

The only significant public building of these years was the Corn Exchange (1861–62), built behind the Town Hall, so that only its interior really counted. It was the last Oxford work of S. L. Seckham, and its polychrome brickwork, iron columns, and carving by O'Shea showed that he was abreast of taste. Even commercial buildings were now Gothic: by far the grandest was the Randolph Hotel, proudly occupying the prominent site opposite the Taylorian and Randolph Building, beside the Martyrs' Memorial. Its vast and symmetrical yellow-brick pile was very characteristic of its architect, William Wilkinson, son of a Witney builder. His accomplishment is shown by his appointment as overseeing architect to the St John's College Estate in North Oxford, and by the praise accorded to him by Viollet-le-Duc, who illustrated five of his houses in his *Habitations Modernes*.[16] Wilkinson also built a splendid new shop in Cornmarket Street for the grocers Grimbly, Hughes and Dawe (1864): the Little-wood's which replaced it in 1964 is no sort of consolation for its loss. A London firm, F. and H. Francis, built grand and fancy premises in the High Street for the London and County Bank (now National Westminster) in 1866. Not to be outdone by the architects, the local builder George Wyatt built himself a new shop and house in St Giles in 1869, proudly claiming that it was all of stone and that his workmen had been involved in the work in a thoroughly medieval spirit. As late as 1880, the Post Office in St Aldate's was Gothic too (by the official architect E. G. Rivers).

Right from the start, Keble attracted a good deal of unfavour-able criticism, from those blinded by ignorance or prejudice. One contemporary who did not like it, but who could not be accused of ignorance, was the eminent historian, and founder of the OSPSGA, E. A. Freeman. He wrote in 1879 to the elder son of the recently deceased Sir Gilbert Scott, with reference to the residential block which his father had built for New College in Holywell Street, between 1872 and 1877, that it was 'of special importance, as the return to plain English and common sense in Oxford buildings, after so many years of Ruskinian tomfoolery'.[17] Scott's work has itself been adversely criticised, largely for its bulk, though it was the College that obliged him to add an extra storey, but Freeman obviously liked the use of stone and a style which takes its cue from Wykeham's original buildings.

Scott's name is associated, more than any other, with the controversial subject of 'restoration', and it was inevitable that Oxford buildings, for better or worse, should undergo the process. Churches and chapels were substantially rearranged and refitted, and the work of the previous century (for example, that of James Wyatt at New College and Magdalen, and that of Sir James Thornhill at All Souls) was replaced with something more 'correct'. Scott's own work – at St Mary the Virgin, New College, Christ Church Cathedral and elsewhere – was mostly first-rate.

Freeman had commended Scott's work at New College for being 'English', and the return to English models was characteristic of architecture throughout the country from the 1870s. The three most important architects working in Oxford in this period were prominent in the movement. All were pupils of Scott. Thomas Graham Jackson, a Wadham man, held a Fellowship there from 1864 until 1880. George Frederick Bodley and Thomas Garner had worked in partnership in London since 1869. A competition was held in 1874 for a new bell-tower over the hall staircase at Christ Church: Jackson's monster tower lost out to a less assertive proposal by Bodley and Garner, but unfortunately the great lantern they designed to go on top was never executed.

However, Jackson's chance came with the commission, in 1876, to design new Examination Schools for the University on a prominent site in the High Street, previously occupied by the city's chief inn, the Angel. The scheme, which itself was a notable symptom of the expansion of the University, went back to 1859, and was intended to provide purpose-built rooms for examinations and lectures, while freeing the ground floor of the Schools Quadrangle for use by the

Bodleian Library. The business of choosing an architect was absurdly mismanaged, but Jackson's design was liked because it was 'in harmony with the existing Schools'. He himself said: 'before my eyes seemed to come the haunting vision of Elizabethan and Jacobean work, and especially of those long mullioned and transomed windows at Kirby Hall in Northamptonshire'.[18] Despite their grim purpose, the Schools have generally found favour, though the critics have been less kind: H.S. Goodhart-Rendel, for example, dismissed them as 'the general public's idea of a work of architecture', and an example of the 'vicious picturesque so common at Oxford'.[19] Certainly no one has ever had much to say for their planning, and they cost the University dearly: in 1875 a limit of £50,000 was set, but by 1882 expenditure had risen to £108,000, and the final cost was nearer £180,000.[20]

An innovation made by Jackson which was to be as influential as his style was his use of stone from Clipsham in Rutland: its durability ensured that it was to become the most used stone in Oxford for decades to come. Bodley had thought of using the 'Renaissance style' for the Schools competition, but was dissuaded by Jackson (before he decided to use it himself). He did, however, use a late sixteenth-century style for the Master's Lodging at University College, built between 1877 and 1880. This very handsome building is too little known.

Jackson's success with the Schools, and his Oxford connections, ensured him a steady flow of commissions for college work, so that his mark was firmly set upon Oxford. At Brasenose, his new front on the High Street was late Gothic in style, to suit the date of the College: for this rather showy work, he used the mixture of coarse stone-rubble walling and Clipsham dressings (apparently first used by him for the High School for Boys), which both he and other architects well into this century favoured, presumably because it gave the effect of instant antiquity. At Trinity, for his irregular 'Front Quadrangle' – arguably his best work in Oxford – he used his Schools Jacobean style. His most extensive work was for Hertford College, where he filled in the gap between Garbett's old Magdalen Hall blocks with a new hall, at first-floor level over the main entrance, built a chapel, better in detail than overall effect, and finally linked his gabled block south of New College Lane with the rest of the College by means of the pretty but underused bridge.

The pace of building by the colleges rose astonishingly towards

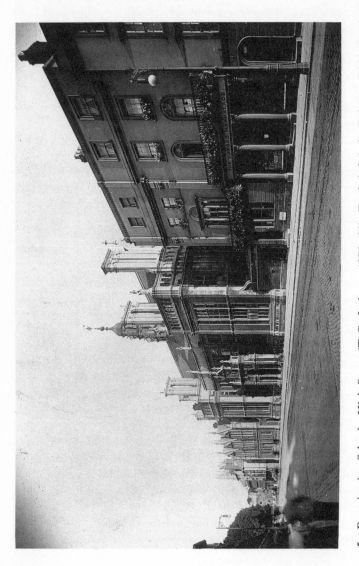

5 Examination Schools, High Street (T. G. Jackson, 1876–82). To their left the Delegacy of Unattached Students, now Ruskin School of Art (T. G. Jackson, 1886–8). *Oxfordshire Photographic Archive*

and around the turn of the century: they were expanding, and it was considered desirable (though no longer required by statute) to house as many undergraduates in college as possible. So, for example, St John's built a new front to the St Giles, in two stages (1880–81 and 1899–1900), the second after the death of the architect, George Gilbert Scott jun. whose restrained but subtle design makes an instructive comparison with Jackson's at Brasenose. What were widely regarded as the best new college buildings in Oxford were built by Magdalen as a result of a limited competition won by Bodley and Garner. Their St Swithin's Quadrangle (1881–85) takes its style from the College itself, and uses it with extraordinary sensitivity and charm. It was even admired by William Morris.

Another excellent architect who did much work in Oxford was Basil Champneys. He continued Scott's range on Holywell Street, on a lower scale and with delightfully pretty detailing, and built an attractive new quadrangle, open to the gardens, for Merton. It is less easy to feel fond of his new High Street front for Oriel, or the new Warden's Lodging for Merton, the most gross of several examples of the demand by heads of houses for vast residences. Both of these were in Renaissance style. Champneys also worked for two of the women's colleges which were newcomers to the Oxford scene. He had designed the first building for Newnham College, Cambridge, in 1874, in the newly fashionable style misleadingly called 'Queen Anne', in red brick with white-painted woodwork. As a result, he was commissioned in 1880 to design the first new building for Lady Margaret Hall, in the same style. Like Keble, it has rooms opening off corridors, an arrangement Champneys (and others) thought appropriate for women's colleges, though not for men's. Champneys also designed a library for Somerville, although the first architect used by that College (in 1881) was Jackson.

Champneys's Oxford masterpiece was, however, in Gothic and in stone: this was one of the two denominational colleges which moved to Oxford. Mansfield, a Congregational foundation, decided to move from Birmingham in 1885, and Champneys designed a picturesque range with a large chapel at one end, and at the other the superb library, whose interior resembles a medieval timber barn. Nearby is Manchester College, where the Unitarians made a less fortunate choice in the elderly Manchester architect Thomas Worthington.

The growth and diversification of the University brought with them a great variety of challenging commissions for architects. One of these again went to Champneys – the Indian Institute, closing the view down the Broad. For it he ingeniously mixed Indian details into his Renaissance style. The development of organised sports demanded buildings, and the commission for a cricket pavilion in the Parks went to Jackson. He was also responsible for two of the several college barges designed by architects associated with their colleges. The Parks, already used for recreation since at least the seventeenth century, had been bought by the University from Merton in 1853, primarily to provide a site for the new Museum, and they had been laid out in the 1860s to a scheme devised by James Bateman, FRS, of Magdalen, best known for his garden at Biddulph Grange in Staffordshire. Unfortunately the success of the Museum in establishing the study of science at Oxford meant that the new buildings required were sited around it. Some were actually attached to it, including Deane's Physics Laboratory, to its north-west (1867 – 69), and the Pitt-Rivers Museum (1885 – 86), while others were detached, such as the Observatory, to its east, by Charles Barry jun. (1874 – 75). This continual encroachment has sadly compromised one of the few amenities made available by the University to the public in general.

This prosperous period also saw the city at last acquiring some buildings of substance and distinction. The two High Schools were both designed by Jackson, showing how much his work was reckoned to be in tune with Oxford. The Boys' School in George Street (1880 – 81) was in stone, in the Jacobean manner which Betjeman christened 'Anglo-Jackson', while the Girls' School in Banbury Road (1879 – 80) was in the 'Queen Anne' style, considered more feminine, with pretty terracotta trim. The plum city job was for a new town hall, to include a library and magistrates' courts, and to cover such a large site that it involved the demolition not only of the old Town Hall but of the Corn Exchange and several other buildings. A competition in 1892 was won by Henry Thomas Hare, a Paris-trained architect new to the city. He produced a building of which it can be proud, though the elaborate ornamentation of its Jacobean style ('in Sir Thomas Jackson's manner, and even more in the manner than Sir Thomas himself', as Betjeman said[21]) is not characteristic of his best work. The excellent planning of its practical and enjoyable interior could never have been matched by Jackson. For its new Corn Exchange and Fire Station, in George Street (1894 – 95), the city went to the local man Henry Wilkinson Moore, who used his standard mildly Jacobean style in brick and stone.

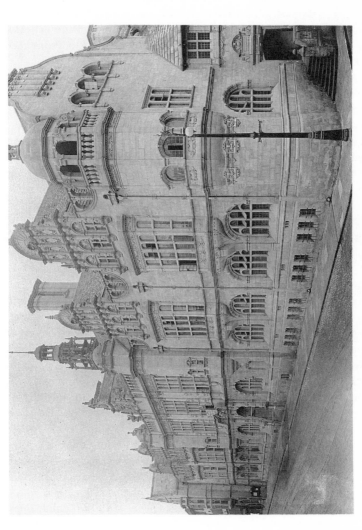

6 Town Hall and former Public Library, St Aldate's (H. T. Hare, 1893–97). *Oxfordshire Photographic Archive*

Sadly, a wonderful opportunity was missed when, at the time of the demolition of St Martin's Church at Carfax in 1896, Hare prepared a superb scheme for remodelling its remaining tower and designing new buildings to flank it.[22] Although the tower was of no architectural interest, antiquarian prejudice ensured that Jackson got the job of completely 'restoring' it, and the only parts of Hare's scheme executed were the buildings on either side of it. The other corners of Carfax were eventually rebuilt, the north-east one by Stephen Salter between 1900 and 1901 ('it shows the consequences of seeing too much Jackson about every day', wrote Pevsner), and the southern ones by Ashley and Newman in restrained 1930s manner (1930 – 31).

Another excellent choice of architect was made by the City when it required three new schools at the turn of the century. Leonard Stokes was not only one of the most talented designers of his time but, as the son of a distinguished inspector of schools, an expert on school design. The three schools he built in Oxford have not been treated as well as they deserve. The only one still used for its original purpose, East Oxford School in Union Street (1899 – 1900), has been much altered (apart from the delightful Infants' School), while the former Central Boys' School on Gloucester Green (also 1899 – 1900), carefully designed to harmonise with humble neighbours, is now stranded in the middle of a large-scale commercial development. By a tragic irony, the Central Girls' School in New Inn Hall Street (1901) has been taken over by St Peter's College, which has been allowed to demolish the rear half, despite its being a listed building.

Around the turn of the century Oxford was fortunate to acquire several other first-rate works of leading architects. G. F. Bodley build the superbly austere church for Father Benson's Society of St John the Evangelist (the 'Cowley Fathers') in Iffley Road: its masterly tower was added in 1902. In Cowley itself Bodley's pupil J. N. Comper built in 1906 a chapel for St John's Home which is simple outside, but a gorgeous recreation of Perpendicular Gothic glory within. Sadly Comper's church for New Hinksey, also dedicated to St John, and begun in 1900, was never completed. Another ecclesiastical genius was Temple Moore, who won the limited competition for Pusey House, an institution intended to commemorate the Catholic ideals of E. B. Pusey, which occupied a prominent site in St Giles. Moore rose to the challenge with a chapel whose quietly understated design is a masterpiece: 'I do not think there is in Oxford any better specimen of Gothic design, old or new', wrote Goodhart-Rendel.[23] Several other ecclesiastical buildings, for the various denominations, went up in these years, but the only other one of outstanding merit was the little Roman Catholic church of SS Gregory and Augustine, built at the top of Woodstock Road in the grounds of a house called Apsley Paddox in 1911. The house was extended by the same architect, Ernest Newton: he was one of the best house architects of the time, and the church has a delightfully domestic atmosphere.

Some of the colleges made good choices of architect from those who were, like Newton, raising the standard of English domestic architecture to its fine Edwardian flowering. Lady Margaret Hall went to (Sir) Reginald Blomfield, nephew of Sir Arthur: between 1896 and 1926 he built a series of blocks in handsome Georgian style. St Hugh's went to a partnership representative of the first-rate architects of Birmingham, Herbert Tudor Buckland and William Haywood, for their comfortable brick buildings (1914–16). Somerville chose the brother of the President of its Council. Little known because their architect died in the First World War, Edmund Fisher's Maitland Building (1910–11) and Hall (1912–13) are unassertive but admirable. One of several other colleges which went to architects connected with their institutions was Magdalen: Edward Prioleau Warren, brother of the President, also worked for Balliol and St John's, and did some work in the town, including the Eastgate Hotel and the Victoria Clock Tower on the Plain. However, not all the building done in these years was of such high quality. For example, Jesus College has its new front in Ship Street designed by R. England, the College Surveyor, in an almost comically 'traditional' style (1906–12), while the Union Society, abandoning its previous record for adventurous patronage, went to the Banbury firm of Mills and Thorpe for their new wing (1910–11).

Surprisingly little building of any importance took place in Oxford within the ten years after the end of the First World War. Two exceptions, side by side in St Giles, were the completion of Pusey House to a modified version of Temple Moore's design by his son-in-law Leslie Moore (1921–26), and Blackfriars, a rather bland work by the Salisbury architect Doran Webb. A London architect, Christopher Wright, built seventeen excellent houses which filled most of the remaining gaps in the north-east corner of the St John's estate in North Oxford.

However, towards the end of the decade, a period of intense activity set in. Little significant work was done by local men. An exception was H. S. Rogers, pupil of and successor to J. T. Micklethwaite of London: he designed a new block for Somerville (1927), and also St Luke's at Cowley (1937–38): this accomplished church has been insufficiently appreciated, partly because of its unpopularity, since it was built by Lord Nuffield at a time of low wages. Nuffield's commercial activities made no worthwhile architectural contribution to Oxford. His first car factory occupied, in 1912, the premises of the former Oxford Military College at Temple Cowley: the cars were made in the three-storey wing built to the design of T. G. Jackson between 1877 and 1878.[24]

The first important outsider in this period was Sir Giles Gilbert Scott, grandson of Sir Gilbert. He had been unsuccessful in the Pusey House competition, but from 1928 to 1930 made a success of the difficult job of carrying on Bodley and Garner's work at Magdalen. His work for Lady Margaret Hall, rather less ingratiating, included a large residential block (1931), and a chapel in the Byzantine style. His major commission was fraught with difficulties. This was the New Bodleian Library, regarded as essential if the library were to remain on its ancient site and not (as at Cambridge) move to a new one. A group of attractive old houses had to be demolished, and a very large building designed in such a way as to disguise its bulk and harmonise with a varied set of neighbours. Scott's work has never been popular, and its careful planning and handsome interiors have been compromised by rapidly changing demands of the Library, but it deserves more appreciation than it has received so far.

Even more active at this time than Scott was Sir Hubert Worthington, son of the architect of Manchester College. His work at Oxford – of which he is said to have been more proud than of any elsewhere – covers over twenty years, starting in 1932 with his extension to Jackson's Radcliffe Science Library. His style was a kind of Art-Deco classical: Pevsner considered that it 'probably derived from that arsenal of the *moderne*, the Paris exhibition of 1925'. His work included the new building for St Catherine's Society (1936), the New College Library (1937–38), the Rose Lane Buildings for Merton (1939), and the Forestry Building (1947–50). He also carried out extensive works of restoration and renovation at the Bodleian Library. It was surprising, in view of Worthington's success, that it was not to him but to the firm of Lanchester and Lodge that the University turned

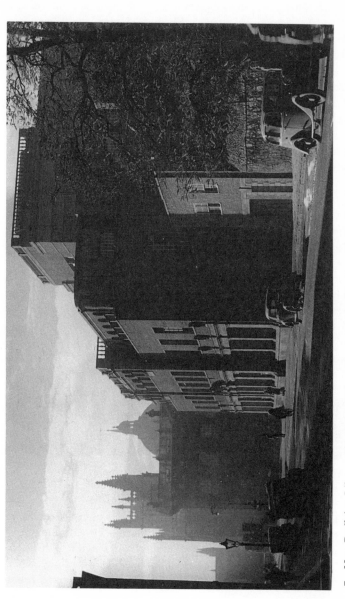

7 New Bodleian Library (Sir Giles Gilbert Scott, 1936–40), from Parks Road, with Clarendon Building, Bodleian Library and Radcliffe Camera beyond. *Oxfordshire Photographic Archive*

for a master plan to try to sort out the muddle and confusion of the 'Science Area'.[25] This was no doubt because they were distinguished planners, but it was a pity that their architecture was so blank and unlovable. Their Inorganic Chemistry Laboratory (which unforgivably involved the demolition of the 'Museum House' by Woodward) was not completed until 1960.

Buildings of the 1930s by other architects were a mixed bag. Finest of all was Campion Hall, the private hall designed for the Jesuits by Sir Edwin Lutyens (1933–36): he ingeniously incorporated an old house, and his first-floor chapel is one of the most striking and effective interiors in Oxford. Its pews are based on those in the seventeenth-century chapel of Rug, which he had seen on a walking tour of North Wales in 1888 with Herbert Baker. Baker's own contribution to the University, Rhodes House (1929), shows his inferiority, with its daft conjunction of a midget Pantheon (with zimbabwe bird on top) and a Cotswold manor house. Other London architects did better: for example, Sir Edwin Cooper's handsome library block for St Hilda's (1932), and Herbert Read's rather tame Rector's Lodging for Lincoln (1929–30). Goodhart-Rendel much admired the new entrance front at Somerville by Percy Morley Horder (1933). However, the Oxford works of the Glasgow architect Thomas Harold Hughes are somewhat disappointing: the best is his Taylorian Institute extension of 1932. Architects too easily lapsed into an effete and dead neo-Georgianism, exemplified by Somerville College Chapel (Courtney Theobald, 1935), the Police Station in St Aldate's (H. F. Hurcombe, 1936), or the Longwall Annexe of Magdalen (J. E. Thorpe, 1935). The Morris Garages in St Aldate's (now Crown Courts; H. F. Smith, 1932–33) have marginally more guts. Presumably the problem was the perennial one – the preference, in a daunting setting, for the safety of 'good taste'. Full-blooded 1930s 'Art Deco' was little seen in Oxford, though a notable exception (even there barely affecting the plain exterior) was the New (now Apollo) Theatre (W. and F. R. Milburn, 1933–34).

When building resumed again after the Second World War, it was on much the same lines as before, which was inevitable since so many of the projects were either completions of earlier buildings or executions of designs made earlier. So the majority of new university buildings in the 1940s and 1950s were by Worthington, Lanchester and Lodge, or Sir Edward Maufe, all looking dreadfully out of date to those who had felt what then seemed the freshening breeze of the Modern Movement. Nowhere can this be better sensed than in *New Oxford*, a booklet produced in 1961 by the undergraduates of the Oxford University Design Society. To them, the ultimate horror was Nuffield College, designed in 1939, but only built between 1949 and 1960. This foundation was to be the chief memorial to Lord Nuffield, and was to have a modern purpose – postgraduate research, especially in the social studies. Christopher Hobhouse, who loathed the idea, at least welcomed the choice of 'Mr Austen Harrison, the excellent architect formerly retained by the Palestine Government'.[26] However, Nuffield's own aesthetic timidity ensured that Harrison's remarkable Siculo-Norman design had to be watered down into something 'in conformity ... with the best tradition of Oxford architecture'.[27] To the authors of *New Oxford*, the result was 'Oxford's biggest monument to barren reaction'. It became fashionable to mock ('the flèche was weak', and so on), but it is interesting to observe that the same publication's prediction, that 'it can only mellow with time, gradually changing from bane to joke', is not being fulfilled. Even Pevsner 'proposed forgiveness' for the tower – 'it has enough identity to be sure that one day it will find affection' – and the history of its design occupies eleven pages of Howard Colvin's *Unbuilt Oxford* (1983).

The buildings that found favour with the authors of *New Oxford* were few enough, but included several in the Science Area by the then official architects, Ramsey, Murray, White, and Ward: some of these, such as the Dyson Perrins Extension (1957 – 59), now have a charmingly period air, but others, such as the eight-storey Biochemistry Building and the nine-storey Engineering Building (both 1960 – 62) are widely unloved. It is curious to recall that at this date high buildings were considered so inevitable that the City Planning Committee approved a policy by which they were to be restricted to this part of the town. This policy was justified on the strange ground that the Keble Chapel was already a high building: the University must have been delighted that Keble just happened to be next to the Science Area, but the sad result has been that the Engineering Building looms, not only over the Parks, but even over the great quadrangle of Keble.

There were fewer college buildings to impress, but the tiny infill at Brasenose by Powell and Moya (1959 – 61), the so-called 'beehive building' at St John's (1960), by Michael Powers of the Architects' Co-Partnership, and the Logic Lane building for University College by Robert Matthew and Johnson-Marshall (1960–61) were all accorded lavish praise. So too was the Law Library, by Sir Leslie Martin and Colin St John Wilson (1961–64), which for Pevsner recalled 'the splendour of Persepolis'. Most exciting of all was the complete new St Catherine's College, begun in 1960 to the design of the Dane Arne Jacobsen. To Pevsner this was 'a perfect piece of architecture', and its elegance did much to secure the triumph of the modern movement in Oxford.

It has to be said, however, that this triumph was assisted by the rather feeble quality of the more traditional buildings going up in Oxford. The most striking were by Raymond Erith: his Provost's Lodging for Queen's (1958–59) has real panache, but his front quadrangle for Lady Margaret Hall, begun in 1957, is not a success. A local architect representing the tail end of the Cotswold Arts and Crafts school was Thomas Rayson, but his neo-vernacular block at Mansfield is very tame, and his completion of the north wing at Keble is dismal.

The 1960s are now regarded as having been the lowest point, not only for architectural quality, but also for the destruction of historic buildings and townscape. A depressing forerunner in both respects was the destruction of the Clarendon Hotel, basically sixteenth-century, to make way for a new Woolworth's, to a design by Sir William Holford (later Lord Holford), which has never pleased anybody much (1956–57). Final permission for this barbarity was given by Harold Macmillan, then Minister of Housing: Oxford never forgave him. Another good building on a prominent site that went was a picturesque house of 1889 by the fine local architect Clapton Crabb Rolfe, at the corner of Broad and Trul Streets: its replacement for Exeter College, completed in 1964, was later described by its own architect, Lionel Brett, as 'pusillanimous and dull'.[28] His explanation for this, that 'Oxford gave me stage-fright', can account for much else in recent years. Balliol College, across the road, having funked the demolition and rebuilding of its main front (planned as part of the celebrations for its seventh centenary), settled for spoiling the work of Salvin and Waterhouse in the Garden Quadrangle instead. New College gave Oxford one its least popular buildings – the Sacher Building, grossly out of place among the small-scale vernacular of Longwall Street, to which it rudely turns its unlovely backside (David Roberts, 1961–62). Equally hated has been the Waynflete Annexe of Magdalen, which replaced a charming Regency house beside the east end of the Magdalen Bridge with a gruesomely banal block (Booth, Ledeboer, and Pinckheard, 1960–61). The city itself was responsible for the wholesale clearance of St Ebbe's. The dreadful Westgate Shopping Centre and multi-storey car park (1969–72) were only too typical of their period. North Oxford began to suffer erosion on an alarming scale: houses in the Woodstock and Banbury Roads were demolished to make way for blocks of flats, or college annexes, which made no effort to harmonise with the suburb.

However, it is some kind of relief to think how much worse the effects of this dismal period might have been. The outstanding boon was the abandonment in 1968 of the longstanding project for a road across Christ Church Meadow, followed by the Council's decision in 1972 not to build any major new roads in the city centre.[29] As part of the 1960s road scheme, Gloucester Green was to have been the site of the largest multi-storey car park in the world. Jericho, due to go the way of St Ebbe's, was reprieved in time for most of it to survive. Conservation Areas ensured that the destruction of North Oxford came to a halt, though infilling and extensions have continued to erode its character. It seems extraordinary now to reflect that in the 1970s the University expected to clear the whole of the 'Keble triangle' (between Banbury and Parks Roads), and also the area west of it between the Banbury and Woodstock Roads, in order to expand the Science Area.

In general Oxford has not been fortunate in recent years in its local architects, but the main jobs continued, until the 1980s, to go to London firms. The results have not been especially inspiring, particularly since colleges have tended to follow fashion in choosing architects who have often been less than enthusiastic about the ensuing commissions. It is noteworthy how often architects whose first buildings in Oxford have been acclaimed as masterpieces have followed them up with less successful ones. For example, Powell and Moya's Wolfson College is redeemed from bleakness only by its riverside setting, and Leslie Martin's ungainly Zoology Building in South Parks Road has none of the Law Library's stylishness. Similarly, Richard MacCormac's more recent Sainsbury Building at Worcester seems unlikely to be matched in quality by his rather bizarre new project for St John's. Other distinguished contemporary architects hardly show at their best in Oxford. James Stirling's Florey Building for Queen's, hidden away in St Clement's, is sought out by architectural students, but is loved neither by its residents nor by local people. Sir Philip Dowson's work (Ove Arup and Partners) at Somerville, St John's, in the Science Area, and at the University College Annexe in North Oxford, is sadly unsympathetic. The work of Howell, Killick, Partridge, and Amis, at St Anne's and St Antony's, is equally unneighbourly, while the extraordinary addition to Keble by Ahrends, Burton and Koralek, for all its sculptural qualities, can scarcely be praised as either economical or practical, and its desert fortress design carries the ideology of the inward-looking quadrangle to freakish lengths. The huge John Radcliffe Hospital, whose white-tiled bulk now looms from Headington Hill over distant views of Oxford, is entirely utilitarian (Yorke, Rosenberg and Mardall, begun in 1968).

Something which essentially changed the appearance of Oxford was the campaign financed by the Oxford Historic Buildings Fund, which between 1957 and 1974 collected £2.4 million towards the cost of refacing and repair.[30] There can be no denying that most of the work had to be done, but the resulting wholesale loss of the texture of antiquity (however spurious much of it may have been) upset many people. It would certainly have grieved Ruskin and Morris.

The current trend towards 'contextual' and historicist architecture is bound to have an appeal for architects designing for Oxford. Two examples under construction are a large block for St Hugh's, which promises to be a grossly over-inflated and poorly detailed parody of its North Oxford neighbours, and a Lodging for the Principal of Manchester College which will provide him with a portico sheltering a balcony on which he can make ceremonial appearances.

A notable feature of recent years has been the loss of many of the City's best buildings to the University. These include three parish churches: St Peter-le-Bailey became the chapel of St Peter's College, while All Saints (formerly the City Church) and St Peter-in-the-East underwent radical internal alteration to serve as libraries for Lincoln College and St Edmund Hall respectively. Both of Jackson's High Schools now belong to the University, along with Stokes' Central Girls' School (see above). Furthermore, to all intents and purposes, the whole area of the city centre east of Turl Street is a university ghetto. Some would argue that this is not only inevitable but right. After all, Pevsner argued in 1974 that 'the ideal firmly to be envisaged ought to be Oxford as the Latin Quarter of Cowley', though he did immediately qualify this as a 'note of flippancy'.[31] The decline of the Cowley car factories adds a new irony to his words.

Notes

The themes of this chapter are developed further in the author's 'Architecture 1800–1914' in the forthcoming Volume VII of *The History of the University of Oxford*. The principal sources for Oxford architecture are *The Buildings of England: Oxfordshire*, by Jennifer Sherwood and Nikolaus Pevsner (Harmondsworth, 1974), and the *Victoria County History* volumes on the University (III, 1954) and the city (IV, 1979), especially the chapter 'Modern Oxford: A history of the city from 1771', by C.J. Day. Other important works not cited in the notes are W.J. Arkell, *Oxford Stone* (London, 1947), and Jennifer Sherwood, *A Guide to the Churches of Oxfordshire* (Oxford, 1989).

1 W. Tuckwell, *Reminiscences of Oxford*, London, 1900, p. 3.

2 Tuckwell, *Reminiscences*, p. 245.

3 Bodleian Library, *Drawings of Oxford by J. C. Buckler, 1811–27*, Oxford, 1951.

4 Alan Crossley (ed.), *Victoria County History of Oxfordshire Vol. IV: The City of Oxford*, London, 1979, pp. 190–1.

5 E. W. Allfrey, 'The architectural history of the College', *Brasenose Quatercentenary Monographs*, I, p. 54, n. 3.

6 P. Howell, 'Newman's church at Littlemore', *Oxford Art Journal*, VI, 1983, pp. 51–6.

7 *Ecclesiologist*, IV, 1845, pp. 32–3.

8 David Prout, ' "The Oxford Society for Promoting the Study of Gothic Architecture" and "The Oxford Architectural Society": 1839–1860', *Oxoniensia*, LIV, 1989, pp. 379–91. The quotation is from p. 380.

9 See Hinchcliffe, below, p. 89.

10 J. Jones, 'The Civil War of 1843', *Balliol College Record*, 1978, pp. 60–8; L. B. Litvack, 'The Balliol that might have been', *Journal of the Society of Architectural Historians*, XLV, 1986, pp. 358–73.

11 P. Howell, 'Samuel Lipscomb Seckham', *Oxoniensia*, XLI, 1976, pp. 337–47.

12 See Hinchcliffe, below, p. 95.

13 P. Howell and I. Sutton (eds.), *The Faber Guide to Victorian Churches*, London, 1989, p. 99.

14 Bodleian Library, MS English Letters e. 28, f. 114, letter of B. Jowett to T. Woolner.

15 A. Saint, 'Charles Buckeridge and his family', *Oxoniensia*, XXXVIII, 1973, pp. 357–72.

16 A. Saint, 'Three Oxford architects', *Oxoniensia*, XXXV, 1970, pp. 53 – 102. See Hinchcliffe, below, pp. 92 – 5.

17 Quoted by Gervase Jackson-Stops in J. Buxton and P. Williams (eds), *New College, Oxford, 1379 – 1979*, Oxford, 1979, p. 263, n. 39.

18 B. H. Jackson (ed.), *Recollections of Thomas Graham Jackson*, London, 1950, p. 134.

19 *Architect and Building News*, CXLIV, 1935, p. 348 (reprinting one of his Slade Lectures).

20 R. Wilcock, *The Building of the Oxford University Examination Schools*, Oxford, 1983.

21 J. Betjeman, *An Oxford Univeristy Chest*, London, 1938, p. 172.

22 Illustrated in *The Builder*, LXXI, 14 November 1896, pp. 403 – 4.

23 *Architect and Building News*, CXLV, 1936, p. 110.

24 B. Johns and J. Wilding, *Nuffield Press*, Oxford, 1985.

25 T. A. Lodge, 'The future of the Oxford science buildings', *Oxford*, Special Number, February 1937, pp. 57 – 9.

26 C. Hobhouse, *Oxford*, London, 1939, p. 115.

27 H. Colvin, *Unbuilt Oxford*, London, 1983, p. 174.

28 L. Brett, *Ourselves Unknown*, London, 1985, p. 160.

29 R. Newman, *The Road and Christ Church Meadow*, Minster Lovell, 1980. See also Scargill, below, pp. 120 – 5.

30 W. F. Oakeshott (ed.), *Oxford Stone Restored*, Oxford, 1975.

31 J. Sherwood and N. Pevsner, *Oxfordshire*, Harmondsworth, 1974, p. 73.

Landownership in the city: St John's College, 1800 – 1968

The colleges of Oxford and Cambridge have in the past been largely dependent on their endowment lands for their prosperity. These were for the most part agricultural lands, but might include urban property which increased revenue when the land became ripe for building. Although a good return could be obtained from urban property, especially during the nineteenth century at the time of town expansion, it could also be more difficult to manage than farmland because of the volatility of the market. Added to this were the restrictions dating from the sixteenth century which had been imposed on the colleges to prevent them jeopardising their long-term commitments and which hampered their full participation in the urban market. Nevertheless, the competition for land in and around the towns during the nineteenth century pushed colleges with town holdings to enter the unfamiliar world of building development.

Shortly after their foundation, St John's College in Oxford acquired about 500 acres immediately to the north of the city. For nearly three centuries this land provided a useful suburban space for pasture and market gardens, but as will become clear pressure to build increased as the nineteenth century proceeded. Progress was slow, however, because as well as the regulations hampering the College's immediate development of the suburb of North Oxford, the social structure of the university city delayed the formation of the sophisticated network of borrowing and lending necessary for the building industry to operate successfully. Another factor impeding the rapid development of North Oxford was the character of the College which required that decisions be made communally and only gradually did a professional bursary emerge to manage the suburban development. The leisurely pace adopted by the College in conducting its business may have led some to assume that the fellows eschewed completely a commercial attitude, but it must be remembered that it was always the College's long-term needs which determined the management of their estates. During the twentieth century, when changes in both the city and the University and in the legislation governing house property put pressure once more on the College, they could only attempt to steer a course which would guarantee the value of their endowment.[1]

Because of the quasi-ecclesiastical nature of the colleges, their endowments were essential to their existence. Although many colleges had medieval origins, they owed their modern foundation to the years immediately following the political and social upheavals of the sixteenth century. Their main purpose at this time was to train the clergy for the newly reformed Church, but despite this ecclesiastical function, the colleges enjoyed the generosity of many secular benefactors who endowed their foundations, mostly with agricultural land, and also on occasion with urban property. In 1874, when the Universities Commission reported on the property held by the universities and colleges, Christ Church of all the Oxford colleges possessed the largest acreage at 29,959, while Pembroke with 1,269 had the smallest. St John's' property comprised 10,429 acres which, compared to the holdings of other colleges, came within the middle range.[2]

St John's College had been founded in 1555 by Sir Thomas White, a London cloth merchant and active member of the Merchant Taylors' Company.[3] He established the College in the buildings of a former Cistercian house of study purchased from Christ Church, and he renamed it after St John the Baptist, patron of tailors. The founder laid down that the College would be composed of fifty fellows and a president, with new fellows recruited from Merchant Taylors' school in London, and schools in Tonbridge, Reading, Coventry, and Bristol, where he had philanthropic interests. In order to support the fifty members, Sir Thomas purchased agricultural land to the west and south of Oxford which produced only about half the income needed. On his death in 1567, Sir Thomas left his London property to his wife and £3,000 to St John's.[4] However, although the College could buy property with this money, the income went to Sir Thomas's wife during her lifetime. When she died in 1572, both the income from their legacy and the London property came to the College and from that date their finances began to improve substantially.

The founder had been anxious that his new College acquire its endowment lands close to Oxford, and besides the buildings for

St John's he had himself bought from Christ Church in 1560 Gloucester Hall and the surrounding closes, lying directly to the west of the city. In 1573 the College purchased about 500 acres, just to the north of the Oxford city wall. St Giles' Fields, as this land was called, had belonged to George Owen, physician to Henry VIII, and St John's bought it from his son for £1,566 13s 4d. This purchase put them in possession of probably the largest single block of land owned by a college in the proximity of Oxford.

As quasi-ecclesiatical institutions the colleges of Oxford and Cambridge were restricted in what they could do with their property. At the time of the religious upheavals during the second half of the sixteenth century, some bishops, finding their revenues eroded, began leasing church property on very long leases. For these they were paid large fees or fines, but those coming after them were then deprived the benefit from the property except for nominal annual rents. In order to counter this practice, legislation was passed to restrict the length of time church property could be leased without renewal.[5] The most common type of ecclesiastical lease became the beneficial lease by which land was leased for twenty years and houses for forty. The annual rent remained low, but when the lease was renewed the tenant paid a fine which usually amounted to one and a half years' notional market value. If the College was to receive the fine only every twenty or forty years this would be poor return on their property, but the lease could be renewed more frequently than that. Leases on land could be renewed for the full term every seven years and leases on houses every fourteen. As the nineteenth century progressed and agricultural prices rose, the beneficial lease system was seen to be archaic and prevented the colleges gaining full advantage of their land, but because it was difficult to extract the college finances from the system, the beneficial leases continued well into the latter part of the nineteenth century.

The beneficial lease system was not conducive to large-scale urban development since the time scale was not long enough for the builder to get his return from the house purchaser. There were other reasons, however, why development around Oxford was slow to take place. First of all the city was surrounded by water, not only by rivers but by water meadows, and had a high water table which tended to cause flooding. In the first half of the century there was some building across Magdalen Bridge in St Clement's, and there was building of small houses, too, in St Aldate's and St Ebbe's in the

south.[6] When depression in the countryside pushed workers into
the city during the 1820s and 1830s, they settled in St Thomas's
parish in the west on land owned by Christ Church, but this land
was low-lying and liable to flood and only poor-quality houses were
built there. Another working-class area called Jericho was built
in the north-west close to the newly-located University Press in
Walton Street. Only the gravel ridge to the north of the city offered
land suitable for the sort of houses expected in a middle-class suburb,
and this was the land owned by St John's, but by mid-century
it was still undeveloped.

R. J. Morris has pointed out that in the early years of the nineteenth
century Oxford's social geography was the opposite of that usually
found in English towns, where the working classes lived in the centre
while the middle classes moved to surrounding suburbs.[7] In Oxford
the suburbs that did appear around the town were inhabited by the
working classes, while the middle classes, even those with a peripheral
interest in the University and the colleges as members of the professions
or tradesmen, preferred to remain in the centre. And of course, the
college fellows were required to reside within the colleges during
term. The regulation, dating from 1561, which prevented fellows
marrying while they retained their fellowships, also meant that
there was little of the inclination found in other towns to establish
a women's sphere in the suburbs as a counterbalance to the increasing
masculinity of the commercial centres.[8] Thus there were a number
of social factors working against the development of a middle-class
suburb in Oxford.

There had been some extension of the town to the north-west of
the city boundary as early as the eighteenth century. On the turnpike
road leading to Woodstock the Radcliffe Infirmary had been built
in 1759 and the Radcliffe Observatory nearby in 1772. Commerce
had come to that side of the city when the Oxford Canal was opened
during the 1790s; later, the Eagle Ironworks was established near
Walton Well in 1825 and in the next year the University Press
removed to Walton Street. These developments, however, remained
isolated and as yet not integrated into the fabric of the town.

Outside the centre of Oxford, too, was Worcester College, which
was founded in 1720 and which occupied the buildings to the west
of the city formerly purchased by Sir Thomas White from Christ
Church. The land to the east and north of Worcester known as
Beaumont and Walton Closes was owned by St John's, and when

Worcester College sought the latter's assistance in laying out a road from their premises to the centre of Oxford, the fellows of St John's began to consider the possibility of developing their land for building purposes.[9] In 1804 St John's agreed to release enough land to make a road from Worcester College in the west to St Giles in the east, but at the same time they also seemed to have decided to take in hand the Beaumont and Walton Closes, and the beneficial leases on the land were not renewed in 1809 and 1811 when they came up for renewal.[10] The College then had to wait another thirteen years until the leases ran out, and it was not until 1822 that they asked Henry Dixon, the College surveyor, to survey the area in preparation for making building leases.[11]

Advertisements for the building land appeared in *Jackson's Oxford Journal* in April 1823.[12] The leases were to be forty-year beneficial leases and the first two plots to be taken were let on the payment of fines of £128 and £117 respectively, with ground rent fixed at £5 per annum.[13] This compares favourably with the fine of 26 guineas previously paid for the whole of the Beaumonts. The houses were to be built in terraces, but under the supervision of the College's surveyor. They had had a drawing made by the architect William Garbett of stone-faced façades for what was to be the north side of Beaumont Street and St John's Street at right angles to it.[14] Although what was built was less dramatic than Garbett's drawing, there was uniformity in the details of the façades which suggests a good deal of control by the College's surveyor. In nearby St Giles, the broad street between St Mary Magdalen and St Giles church, a number of fine stone-faced houses had been built during the eighteenth century, and Beaumont Street and its subsidary streets should be seen as a continuation of this development. The building lots were taken by local tradesmen such as George Kimber, a local tallow merchant, and builders such as George Bennett and John Chaundy.[15] Those who took leases on the houses comprised a cross-section of tradespeople and Beaumont Street, along with St Giles, became the residence of professional men. Another less formal set of terraces was built in Walton Street with chequered brick facades and small front gardens, and these houses were also taken by local tradespeople.

It took some time for all the building lots in Beaumont and Walton Closes to be taken up, and not until the 1840s was the development complete. It is difficult to glean from the Register of St John's College, the record of the meetings of the senior fellows and the president, what the attitude of the fellows was to development, and just when the idea of building a residential suburb in St Giles' Fields occurred to them. In 1825 they asked Dixon to survey their land there, and in October 1827 a notice appeared in *Jackson's Oxford Journal* to the effect that an application would be made in the next session of Parliament to bring in a Bill of Enclosure for the Parish.[16] There was not a large amount of common land in St Giles' Fields, but if development was to take place it was important that the College should be able to take into hand all the available land. The Enclosure Act was finally passed in 1829 and in September that year Dixon, as the commissioner for the enclosure, began to take requests for allotments from the various freeholders and proprietors in the parish.[17]

Dixon also made a valuation in 1829 of the house owned by St John's in St Giles' Field, and discovered a certain amount of irregularity among the leaseholders.[18] An area of the land north of the Radcliffe Observatory was leased by Thomas Tagg, among others, on a twenty-year beneficial lease. Tagg was a market gardener who let out small plots to tenants who were, on investigation, paying him more than he admitted to the College. What was called Tagg's Garden was given a map of its own in the enclosure documents of 1832 and it is evident that the density of building in this area required a map of a larger scale than was necessary for the other parts of the parish which were primarily agricultural in nature.[19] During the 1820s it seems that in Tagg's Garden a number of cottages and other structures were being built outside the control of the College. This practice was stopped in 1842 when the leases fell in and the College began leasing the property again on twenty-year building leases.[20] But the informal development of an area like Tagg's Garden was symptomatic of what happened to a 'working suburb' when its function began to change.

The suburb of St Giles had kept its agricultural character into the nineteenth century, and John Henry Newman could remember when corn was still grown in the parish. By mid-century the land was used mostly for pasture and for market gardens by the local butchers, dairymen, and greengrocers. The suburb was also the chief source of gravel for the town and the site of brickmaking. Besides making space for these utilitarian functions, St Giles' Fields was a place of recreation where games were played and informal sports like fishing pursued. For the reasons given above the call for a great expansion of the town's housing on cheap surrounding agricultural land did not happen at the same time in Oxford as it did in other towns, and it was the threat from other quarters that alerted the fellows of St John's to the dangers of delaying too long in developing their residential suburb, if that was in fact what they intended doing.

One of the threatened changes to the College's property was the introduction of a railway line from Brentford in West London to a terminus on the west side of the suburb of St Giles at Walton Wells. The line would have entered the College's land just south of the present site of Park Town and have effectively cut off the southern third of their estate from the rest of their property. The line was proposed in 1851 by the Oxford, Worcester, and Wolverhampton Railway, a subsidary of the Great Western Railway, and would have meant any plans the College had for a residential estate would have had to take account of the railway and its accompanying appurtenances.[21] Although there were two more occasions when the College's property in St Giles tempted railway companies to contemplate railway lines in the area, these both came to nothing.[22]

One modern function the fellows allowed on their property was the town's cemetery, which was to replace the overcrowded churchyards of Oxford's parish churches. In 1844 the Church Burial Ground Committee approached St John's about buying some of their land for the new cemetery and a site was found near the canal behind the Eagle Ironworks.[23] The Board of Guardians also asked the College for land in St Giles for a new workhouse and this request they were more reluctant to grant. In February 1849 the Board of Guardians was interested in an exchange of land with St John's, but in March of the same year the Guardians agreed to purchase 9 acres on the east side of Banbury Road owned by New College.[24] There were a number of such pockets of land in St Giles' Fields owned by colleges other than St John's as well as by other freeholders. Villa residences had been built on some of these, for example the Mount and the Lawn, two houses across Banbury Road from the site the Guardians had just agreed to buy. But whereas the villas could only enhance the value of the College's property, the building of a workhouse in the locality would result in 'a great depreciation in the Marketable Value of the Lands' as the surveyor, James Saunders, reported to the College in June 1849.[25] Eventually outside circumstances forced the Guardians to drop their plans for the new workhouse, and they decided to see the 9 acres in Banbury Road for house building.

After considering proposals by Samuel L. Seckham and by E. G. Bruton, the Guardians decided to accept Seckham's scheme for middle-class houses on the Banbury Road site.[26] Seckham also offered to buy about a quarter of the land for £2,000 and shortly after he made an offer of £1,200 on another portion of the property where he proposed building a terrace. His scheme for the development, which was to be called Park Town, provided for a mix of terraces, semi-detached houses, and detached villas, placed in such a way on the long, narrow site that a picturesque effect would be created once the central garden and the planting on the Banbury Road had matured.[27] Seckham had the financial backing of his father and uncle, two local men of affairs, and in 1857 he and his backers established the Park Town Company.[28] In order to interest investment, they set up a tontine by which each shareholder nominated one life per share. When the last seven lives were left it was expected that the estate would be complete and then the remaining shareholders would divide up the capital. The company hoped to raise £23,400 on 780 shares, but in the end only 278 were taken up and the company went into liquidation in 1861. Park Town itself was a social success and residents were found to fill the houses, but financially it made no fortunes. That Seckham and his associates felt that they had to resort to a tontine suggests that the means of raising capital in Oxford were at this time still somewhat primitive, and this may have been another reason for a slow start ot middle-class housing developments in the city.

The presence of Park Town must have been an encouragement to St John's to develop their land, as much as the railway and the work-house were an incentive to set their plans in motion before any other outside agent forced development in one direction or another. From Saunders's words in 1849 it does sound as though the College were contemplating some future development, and in 1840 they had decided not to renew the lease on the land in Woodstock Road held by the Duke of Marlborough.[29] The land came to hand in 1853 and shortly after the College asked Seckham to draw up a plan for a housing estate which included large villas facing the main road, smaller semi-detached houses, and a terrace behind, as well as a church.[30] Just at this time the elderly steward of the College, Baker Morrell, retired in favour of his son, Frederic, who seems to have taken the idea of developing the College's suburban property seriously and to have been responsible for forwarding the project during the initial years.

The first obstacle to overcome was the effect of the beneficial leases, and by starting to run them out during the 1840s, the College had in hand by 1856 enough land to start the building process at least from the west side of the Woodstock Road to the Banbury Road north of Bevington Road and south of the present-day Canterbury Road. The other obstacle was the restriction on long leases. The leasehold system which operated on most London estates, whereby the builder took the plot at a nominal rent, built the house and sold the lease to the buyer at a price which covered the building cost and the builder's profit, was very attractive to those involved in the building process. The leaseholder continued to pay the nominal ground rent and, after the period of usually ninety-nine years, the house returned to the ground landlord. The system satisfied all the parties involved since the builder received his profit, the ground landlord had the anticipation of gaining back the site at an enhanced value, and the leaseholder had a property on which he need only pay a small annual rent until more than a lifetime away the property reverted to the ground landlord. As matters stood the option of the long lease was not open to the colleges without a private Act of Parliament, and in 1854 application was made by St John's to parliament for such an act to be passed which it was in August 1855.[31]

Once the obstacles to building had been removed the College went ahead with the lease of the first lots on the west side of Woodstock Road. The result was two semi-detached houses built in the Italianate style of Seckham's Park Town by John Dyne, a London builder. And that was all. Dyne took out his lease in 1856 and mortgaged the property to Morrell, the College's steward, but he soon passed the unfinished houses on in the next year to a local builder, Thomas Winterbourne, who completed them.[32] Why had the project so abruptly come to a halt? It may have had something to do with the lack of capital available in the city for building purposes. The College's first venture into development coincided with the attempts by the Park Town Company to raise money through their tontine. Dyne's lack of local connections may also have made it difficult for him to borrow the necessary money to build his houses.

For any housing development to succeed there was a requirement for a network of lenders and borrowers which builders and house purchasers could use effectively at the different stages of the building process. Besides the banks and local solicitors there were two organisations in Oxford which provided money for building. One was the Oxford and Abingdon Permanent Benefit Building Society, founded in 1851 and run on building society lines.[33] Borrowers were required to become members and themselves had to hold a minimum number of shares in the society. In this way the Society had some control over the borrowers, and their policy that they would lend only on houses already erected meant that they avoided the worst excesses of speculation. The other organisation, the Oxford Building and Investment Company, was established in 1866 and did not require its borrowers to be investors.[34] They were prepared to lend to almost any builder, and although during the good years they were able to pay their investors 8 to 10 per cent interest, when speculation began to run into the ground in the late 1870s, they were extremely vulnerable.

Again we might return to the social composition of Oxford to explain the hesitant start to St John's development. The town at this time had no industry to speak of, and its tradesmen and its professional men depended almost exclusively on the University and the colleges for their business. Although the colleges spent money in the town and the fellows and undergraduates patronised the local shops, their actual wealth lay elsewhere. For example, when a fellow married he was forced to give up his fellowship and to pursue his career outside Oxford, usually in the Church. The savings of the married couple and any money contributed by their families to set up their home would be spent in another part of the country, so that a large part of the resources of the middle-class living in the city never saw Oxford. This had a cumulative effect on the surplus capital there was available in the city for development schemes like St John's North Oxford estate.

The organisation of the College may also have had some influence on the slowness of events. Although they had an advocate of the development in their steward, they did not appoint an estates committee to oversee the special demands of their property, both rural and urban, until 1862.[35] The administration of the College's estates was in the hands of the Senior bursar who, until 1867, was elected yearly from among the senior fellows. Some continuity in the bursary was maintained by virtue of the senior bursar for one year automatically becoming the junior bursar the next. Decisions about the College's estates were taken communally at the scheduled general meeting which occurred in April and October each year, with extraordinary meetings called when circumstances required. If business was not considered urgent it was only dealt with at the next general meeting, and as a result it often took a long time for decisions to be made and implemented. In 1867 it was decided that the burden of work in the bursary required that the bursar should be elected for a five-year period, with the option of continuing in his post for a further five years.[36]

In the autumn of 1859 the fellows appointed a committee to consider how best to proceed with the development of the North Oxford estate, given that it appeared to be stalled with only two houses built.[37] The decision reached was that seven lots on Woodstock Road, and the St Giles' Glebe land at the south end of what was called Norham Manor on the east side of Banbury Road, should be offered for auction in the summer of 1860. The buyers were to bid for the ground rents of the various lots, with the understanding that they would build houses of a type acceptable to the College. These first two auctions did not produce exceptional results and years later John Galpin, a local surveyor, remembered that what he called 'a very low class of people' took the plots and proceeded to remove the gravel and anything else of value before the College could regain possession of their land.[38] The auction did alert the public to the fact that the land was available and, as the 1860s progressed, more individuals took plots and had their own architects build substantial villas there.

At first Seckham was retained as the overseeing architect of the Woodstock Road site, but by the mid-1850s William Wilkinson, another local architect, had taken control of the whole estate.[39] It was up to him to lay out the roads as they were required and it was also his task to approve each application, deciding whether the house was suitable as to style and standard of materials. Wilkinson himself built a number of houses in a robust neo-Gothic style, and during the first twenty years of the development the Gothic prevailed. The College was especially interested in the quality of the materials used and stipulated that the houses be built of brick and stone, without the use of cement or artificial stone. They also demanded that the tenant build a wall around the plot with a low wall to the street.[40] The roads and drains were paid for in the first instance by the College, and then a rate was levied on the leaseholders when enough houses were built and occupied.

The first houses in North Oxford were purpose-built for individuals, mostly tradesmen and a few university professors, a class of academic who had always been allowed to live outside the colleges. In Norham

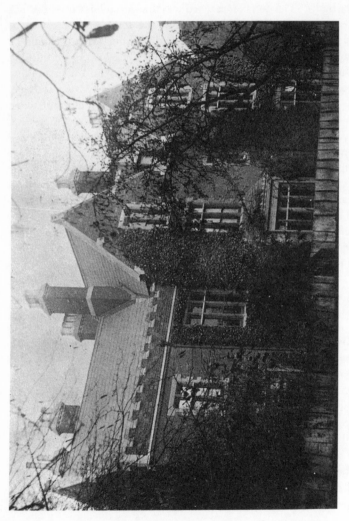

8 The house of Max Mueller (1823–1900), part of the Norham estate of St John's College which was developed from 1860. Mueller held the Chair in Comparative Philology and was the first married fellow of All Souls. *Oxfordshire Photographic Archive*

Manor the first residents were Professors Goldwin Smith and Montague Burrows, soon followed by George Mallam, a local solicitor.[41] In Woodstock Road early houses were built for Edwin Butler, a wine merchant, William Lucy, the owner of the Eagle Ironworks, and Robert Hills, a photographer. While the main part of the estate was laid out in large lots for middle-clas villas, the west side of the estate was reserved for working-class cottages. As early as 1864 the fellows had expressed their intention to build workers' cottages, and this was at least six months before the Great Western Railway proposed moving their carriage-building works from Paddington in London to Oxford.[42] It has been suggested that St John's reacted to the news by laying out plots for cottages. The College did ask Wilkinson in April 1865, shortly after the railway company had announced their intention, to lay out building plots for small houses on their property near Worcester College and in Jericho, but even when the company decided to abandon their plans for the carriage works in Oxford, the College continued to reserve the west side of the estate for working-class houses. By dividing their estate by class, the College was in a better position to control what was built since they could insist that if a builder was not able to afford to build an expensive house in the middle-class area, he take plots in the section reserved for the cottages. In fact the builders were noticeably split between those who worked mainly in the Kingston Road area and those who built the middle-class houses on the rest of the estate.

Towards the end of the 1860s more houses were built speculatively in both the working-class and middle-class sections of the estate. One of the more active developers was the builder and architect, Frederick Codd. He was a native of East Dereham in Norfolk, but he had come to Oxford from London in about 1865.[43] The houses he built are to be found in Banbury Road, Norham Gardens, and Bradmore and Canterbury Roads. He also designed houses in a sturdy Gothic style, with less originality than Wilkinson, but still very acceptable in the context of North Oxford. In order to prevent builders taking plots and then sitting on them without building, the College, in their building agreement, asked that the lease be taken out on the house usually within two years of the building agreement being signed. They also reserved the right to take possession of a house not yet built beyond the first floor if the builder should go into liquidation or bankruptcy.[44] Codd held shares in the Oxford and Abingdon Building Society and in order to lease his houses before the time limit he would sometimes take the leases himself, mortgaging the houses to the society.[45] He was then usually able to sell the leases quite quickly, but as the 1870s advanced the housing market in Oxford began to slow. In 1876 Codd had just built a number of houses in Canterbury Road and his debts to the Oxford and Abingdon Building Society amounted to £16,047, while he still had building commitments in Fyfield and Crick Roads on the Norham Manor estate. In January of that year Codd was advertising the houses in Canterbury Road for sale, but by July he had not yet sold them and had to take six leases himself on houses he then mortgaged to the society. It appeared that the market for the sort of detached villas he was building had dried up, and since the class of house built was determined by the College, he did not have the option to build more cheaply at a higher density. By September Codd's serious debt to the building society forced him into liquidation.[46]

The other speculator who was most active on the estate at this time was John Galpin. He was the secretary of the Oxford Building Investment Company which provided the money for a substantial amount of building in North Oxford, mostly on the west side, where the smaller houses were built. Galpin's own builder, John Dover, borrowed a total of £105,795 from the company over a period of seventeen years.[47] Together Galpin and Dover were especially active in the middle-class areas, including Norham Gardens, Bradmore, Crick, and Norham Roads, and Farndon and Warnborough Roads. At the height of its success the Oxford Building Company drew in funds from hundreds of small local investors, and their ability to attract investment led to their downfall as depression in the housing market took hold. When building came to a halt there was little demand for loans, with the result that the company was not increasing the value of their bondholders' and shareholders' investments. In order to keep business going the company even bought land themselves with the hope of encouraging building to continue over the slump. Desperate to pay their dividends, they borrowed money on the security of leases they held in North Oxford and on other estates. Finally in March 1883, the company accounced that although they had total confidence in the future they were not prepared to pay a dividend.[48] Their confidence was not shared by the public and within a period of two weeks £40,000 had been withdrawn. On 5 April 1883 a petition for winding up the company was filed, and voluntary liquidation followed.

There is not much indication in the minutes of St John's estates committee that these upheavals were taking place in connection with their Oxford property. Whatever happened, they could wait until the market revived, and even as the slump worsened, they were receiving building proposals from a new breed of developer for plots in Southmoor and St Margaret's Roads.[49] Although the College seemed indifferent to the ups and downs of the housing market they were deeply concerned about another depression, the one that was affecting the agricultural markets.[50] From the records, St John's was indeed adversely affected, although part of the problem was that they had become used to larger revenues and had more commitments to the University and to the improvement of their rural property, as they made the transfer from beneficial leases to rack renting. Throughout the nineteenth century one of the themes of reform was the increased contributions the colleges should make to the University so that the level of research and teaching could be raised. The Universities Commission, which reported in 1874 on the property held by the universities and the colleges, was intended to form the basis for deciding the level of the colleges' contributions.[51] In his answers to the Commissioners' questions, the bursar of St John's was very careful not to suggest that their increase in revenue would necessarily allow them to commit themselves to extensive contributions. He was especially cautious about the prospects for the urban property, whose value, he suggested, was subject to fashion.

As it happened the urban property held its value while the agricultural depression bit hard into the College's revenues. The situation became so bad during the 1880s that the College had to reduce the payments to their fellows and scholars and to seek exemption from their commitments to the University. As far as their Oxford property was concerned, the constraint on their finances made the College reluctant to become involved in any extensive road building, and during the slack years at the end of the 1870s and early 1880s they refrained from releasing any more building land in North Oxford, thus contributing to the depression among the local builders.[52]

Despite the agriculture depression, the housing market in Oxford began to pick up again during the 1880s. Once the crash of the Oxford Building Company had been absorbed, building began again in North Oxford, especially in the newly laid-out streets north of St Margaret's Road in the north-west section of the estate. Here Walter Gray, one who was instrumental in the fall of the Oxford Building

Company, was active as developer in collaboration with Wilkinson's nephew, the architect Harry Wilkinson Moore. In 1886 Moore took over the supervision of the estate on his uncle's retirement and continued in this position until 1903. Gray acted as developer and financier, sometimes taking building plots himself, but just as often simply supplying the capital to a small group of local builders.[53] He also provided mortgages for the purchasers of the houses, who were mostly local tradesman from the Walton Street area. These people wanted the houses either to live in or, just as likely, for an investment, and they found that the smaller houses on this part of the estate suited their purposes admirably.

The bursar of St John's made it known that the College wished to reserve the north-eastern section of North Oxford, north of Park Town, for individuals wishing to build their own houses.[54] Purpose-built houses were erected in the Woodstock and Banbury Roads, but the College's reluctance to open what was called the Bardwell estate in the north-eastern section to speculation meant that that was the last area to be developed. Eventually they allowed speculative building there, but the houses were all of a substantial character, distinct from the smaller houses on the west side of the estate.

The College also continued to foster cottage building, making the decision in 1885 to develop land north of Kingston Road near the canal with small housing suitable for the working classes.[55] They had been disappointed that the houses built in Southmoor Road in the early 1880s were too large for working people to afford. The College even tried to build cottages themselves, but they were informed that this was not within their powers, and in the end the Oxford Industrial and Provident Land and Building Society took the plots on the newly laid-out Hayfield Road and built ninety-six cottages there.[56]

By the First World War the suburb of North Oxford was nearly complete. There were still allotments to the north of the Bardwell estate to be built upon, and the top end of Bainton Road in the north-west remained unfinished. At the other end of the estate, many of the houses had been up for forty or fifty years, and the area had assumed an air of stability, enhanced by the presence of mature trees and gardens. Over the years the social composition of the suburb had become more varied, as a greater number of people had access to the new houses. For example, more academic families moved to the area, as the 1877 Universities Act allowed colleges to exercise discretion in the application of the rule governing celibacy among their fellows.[57] Some colleges were liberal on this question and, like Balliol and Merton, allowed some married fellows even before the Act was passed. Others, such as St John's, were more conservative and resisted the change. Even when the fellows were allowed to marry and establish a family in Oxford, if they did not have financial help from their families they were often in no position to rent a house in North Oxford, let alone take the lease on one. The communal life of the colleges meant that the modest pay of the fellows was compensated by their board which they received while resident, and if they were to live outside and to support a respectable middle-class household it was necessary for each college to devise a new structure of pay and the provision of pensions. This took time, but by 1914 at least, North Oxford had become within reach of many academics.

During the nineteenth century, in order to discourage conservative members of the University coming in from the country to vote down reforms, a rule was passed that members of the University Congregation had to reside within a mile and a half of Carfax in the centre of Oxford. As more retired members of the University, especially the clergy, came to live in North Oxford, it was found that a new conservative constituency had formed itself within the boundaries, and around 1913 it was agreed to do away with the residence limitation and to reduce those allowed to vote on changes in the University to those who were immediately concerned with its academic life.[58] This decision, together with the advent of the motor car, meant that the boundaries of what was considered suburban Oxford were greatly extended. This was to have implications for St John's property as the composition of the suburb gradually changed after the war. The policy of the College was to maintain the residential character of the suburb, and if there were applications to make additions to the houses or to change their use, the neighbours affected were to be consulted. As the large houses built for the professors and the wealthy tradesmen lost their appeal to this class of resident, they were divided into flats or let out as rooms, especially to the women undergraduates whose colleges were mostly concentrated in North Oxford. Some of the large houses were taken by the assortment of educational institutions which were drawn to the environs of the University. The residential character of the suburb was, nevertheless, maintained under the watchful supervision of the bursar of St John's.

Between the wars change was also afoot in Oxford at large, although the effects were not fully felt until after 1945. The most dramatic development was the establishment in Cowley of Morris's motor works and the increase in the overall population of Oxford of 20 per cent from 1921 to 1931.[59] The great influx of workers was confined to the new industrial suburb which sprang up in Cowley to the east of the city, but central Oxford began to feel the effects of the growth through a significant increase in traffic. At least from the 1930s traffic became an obsession with the growing numbers of planners who set their minds to the problems of the city centre, and although St John's and its Oxford property were beyond the area for which the schemes were planned, throughout the 1950s and 1960s their North Oxford estate always entered into the schemes as the route north out of the centre.

The other significant change was the expansion of the activities of the University. Once its finances were put on a firm basis after the First World War, the University could develop its various faculties, especially in the sciences. The science area had been established around the Museum in South Parks Road, but as early as 1913, the University approached St John's for a site at the top of the Parks Road for an engineering laboratory.[60] Later in the 1930s they sought to buy the whole of the island site in what became known as the Keble Triangle. This was not fully developed until the 1960s, by which time they had bought more of the College's property in Banbury Road following the recommendations of Lord Holford that the science area expand northwards.[61] Despite these incursions by the University, St John's tried to retain the residential character of North Oxford with varying degrees of success.

After the First World War St John's, along with the other colleges, still relied on their endowment lands for their revenue. In 1920 they chose a bursar from outside the College who had strong agricultural interests and who took an active part in bringing their rural property into profit during a very difficult period for farming.[62] At a time when other investors were moving out of property, they were constrained by the Universities and Colleges Estates Act of 1925, whose purpose was to prevent colleges selling their land and squandering the proceeds in doubtful investments. Whenever they wished to sell land, they had to seek the permission of the Minister of Agriculture who had replaced the Land Commissioner, and he would be entrusted with the money until another piece of land was purchased or some other approved use was found for it. Thus the endowment of the colleges was safeguarded from short-term investment and speculation. The long-term nature of the colleges' investments often gave the impression that they were acting against their commercial interests, for example when St John's refused to allow small terraced houses in areas of their North Oxford estate where houses were not selling and building was slow. On the other hand they could cause confusion and alarm when they acted to further their interests by, for example, raising rents. The truth was that the colleges were neither commercial enterprises nor philanthropic institutions, and followed their own path of necessity.

After the Second World War, the fellows of St John's were faced with a number of decisions connected with the house property in Oxford. The houses that had been let on beneficial leases in the Beaumont Street area and those let on sixty-six-year leases in Jericho and Kingston Road had come into hand and were being rented to the tenants directly by the College.[63] The other area mostly in their direct control was formed by the streets north of the Radcliffe Observatory in what had been Tagg's Garden. This area was now referred to as Walton Manor, and here in the small terraced house the College housed many of their staff. Beaumont and St John's Street they wanted to keep, and Walton Manor was attractive to them not just as accommodation for their staff, but as an area of small and relatively cheap housing in proximity to the centre of Oxford. Much of the other property in their possession was in poor condition, and it was decided that this could well be redeveloped with flats or new houses, and in the meantime it should be rented out under the supervision of a woman housing manager.[64] The other decision which would become more pressing as time passed was what the College should do with the houses on long leases when they began to revert to them in the 1960s. The fate of both the rented and the leased property became more pressing with the threat and eventual passing of the various housing legislation during the 1950s and 1960s.

By the early 1950s the College found that their income was not keeping up with expenditure, and they explored ways of increasing their revenues.[65] While it was suggested that more money could be obtained from their property, it was difficult to see how they could in the near future make more from their Oxford houses. The smaller houses which were within their management were mostly of a type which came under the Rent Restriction Acts, while the houses on long leases would not start coming into their possession for another ten to fifteen years, and up until then they could only expect to receive the ground rent, which was in most cases very small in comparison to the value of the houses. The suggestion was then made that the College would perhaps do well to diversify its assets. In 1958 70 per cent of their external income came from house property and only 8.8 per cent from gilt-edged investments and 1.2 per cent from equities.[66] Until 1964 and a new Universities and Colleges Estates Act permitted colleges to take more responsibility for their own affairs, the College was constrained in how much they could diversify, but the fellows did begin to address the problems arising from their Oxford properties by commissioning a Report on the subject in 1960.[67]

An added incentive to formulate a policy for the Oxford property was that for a number of years there had been rumour that the leasehold system would be reformed so that the holders of long leases could have the right to buy the freehold from their ground landlords. Except for the large estates in London and houses held by corporate bodies such as the colleges, most of the original ground landlords had long since sold their rights. The proposed legislation was intended to discourage unscrupulous speculators from buying up the reversion of leases on the point of expiring, with the intention of evicting without compensation the leaseholders when the leases fell in. The legislation would mean, however, that the College could expect to receive only the current value of the house before dilapidations and without the prerogative to redevelop, which was one of the incentives to let on long leases in the first place. It was unlikely that such a measure would be taken before a Labour government was in power, but since the College had to work in the long term, the bursar asked that they consider the implications such a reform would have, especially for their North Oxford property.

The recommendations of the Report confirmed the College's commitment to keeping their houses in Beaumont and St John's Street and those in the Walton Manor area.[68] The houses north of Park Town and east of Banbury Road still had a number of years to run on their leases, and their value would probably exclude them from any leasehold legislation. The large houses in the Norham Manor area were already of interest to the University for further development and those houses around St Anne's and St Antony's Colleges would probably eventually be purchased by those institutions when their leases expired. Property on the west side of Woodstock Road, it was recommended, should be sold.

As soon as the Report appeared, the College began to consult those involved in the property market, but the advice the fellows received was contradictory and left them more confused than they were before. Although the consensus was that the College was 'sitting on a gold-mine', advice ranged from wholesale redevelopment of North Oxford to doing nothing for the next fifteen to twenty years while the College waited for the leases to fall in. Predictably enough the fellows chose the latter course. However, a number of events outside the College's control determined their eventual course of action. First of all the Rent Restrictions Act of 1965 gave the local rent officer jurisdiction over the level of rents in an area.[69] Although the legislation made provision for rent rises from time to time, landlords could not take advantage of the scarcity value of dwellings in their area. This meant that the College could not hope to increase their revenues through a rise in rents, but were faced with ever-mounting repair costs while rents remained static.

Then in February 1966 the long awaited White Paper on leasehold reform was published in preparation for the passing of the legislation which took place in 1967.[70] This confirmed the College in their decision to sell the houses in Kingston Road, and at the same time they set up a committee to deal with the leasehold legislation. The Leasehold Reform Act was intended to affect only those houses which had a rateable value below £200, but the College received applications from leaseholders of houses of higher value. These applications were treated on their merits, and eventually many houses above the £200 limit were sold. The Leasehold Reform Act stood at the beginning of a long drawn-out process by which St John's gradually sold the freeholds of a large proportion of their Oxford houses, although they still own approximately 200 dwellings, both houses and flats.

That St John's College owned the land immediately to the north of central Oxford goes some way to explaining why such a complete nineteenth-century suburb now exists in North Oxford. As has been seen, there were impediments to the colleges developing their properties, and especially their urban properties. The beneficial lease system and the strictures against long leases prevented St John's laying out their land for building until they had their leased property in hand and they had by private Act of Parliament been empowered to grant ninety-nine-year leases. But part of the slowness in the development of North Oxford was also caused by the social structure of Oxford as a university town in the nineteenth century, where industry was discouraged and a large proportion of the middle classes had no interest in disposing of their capital in the city while they resided within the colleges. It has been assumed that St John's freed their land for building as a reaction to the release from celibacy of the college fellows, but as has been shown, the initial building started a good twenty years before the enabling legislation which gave the colleges the authority to allow their fellows to marry. And it was another ten to twenty years before many of them could afford a house in the suburbs. Perhaps more interesting is the way the conservative policies of the College kept the character of North Oxford as a residential suburb so close to the city centre.

As has been shown, St John's had both to maximise the revenue from its endowment, and to ensure the long-term value of its property. In this it was similar to other colleges and institutions, but because its Oxford property was in such close proximity to the College buildings in St Giles', St John's had a particular interest in the physical and social composition of the suburb. Others with similar long-term interests, such as the Calthorpe family, owners of the Birmingham suburb of Edgbaston, insisted on the high value of property built on their estate and bided their time when the market indicated that houses of a lesser value would sell better than middle-class villas.[71] Because North Oxford was so close to St John's and the other colleges, there was the added incentive to keep strict control over what was built so that there was no danger of the suburb degenerating into a poor, ill-kept district. In this the College was similar to the Foundling Hospital whose Bloomsbury estate was carefully laid out and maintained so that the reputation of the nearby hospital would not suffer.[72] There was a chance in the 1960s that the interests of the College would have best been served by the wholesale redevelopment of their Oxford property, and one argument against this course of action was the opprobrium the College might suffer if they allowed high-density development in an area of the city which through the conservative policies of the College had survived to become a desirable amenity.[73]

Although there was no overall plan for North Oxford, its coherence came from the College's requirement that each section be completed before the others were started and that the social status of the houses be determined by their value. The instrument in this was the estate architect, who worked under the direction of the bursar as the representative of the fellows. During the history of North Oxford the power of the bursar in relation to the fellows varied considerably, and if the institutional organisation of the College could be said to have influenced the way the suburb developed, it could also be said that the process of developing and managing the suburb affected the status and importance of the College's bursary. The most distinctive feature of the College's stewardship of their endowment was the communal responsibility taken by the senior fellows, but increasingly the estates committee and the position of the bursar assumed more importance. When it was decided in 1867 to elect the bursar for a five-year period, the fellows acknowledged that the task of managing the College's estates had grown beyond the general competence. However, it was not until after the First World War that they were able successfully to employ a professional man as bursar. Although the bursar took control of the estates, his underlying role was still one of adviser and executant of the will of the fellows. During the discussions after the Second World War about the future of the College's estates, the suggestion that the College should diversify their investments was initiated among the fellows. Generally, however, the need for consensus tended towards a cautious, conservative policy concerning the College's property, and although St John's no longer owns a large section of residential Oxford, their influence is still to be seen in the suburban streets of North Oxford. By hanging on to the suburb until they were forced to relinquish control by the Leasehold Reform Act, they ensured that North Oxford would survive into a period when nineteenth-century suburbs were once more valued as desirable residential property and, for a time at least, redevelopment could be held at bay. When compared to the other colleges, St John's did not possess the largest endownment, but its effect on the city of Oxford has been the greatest.

Notes

1   My research on the Oxford property of St John's was commissioned by the President and Fellows of St John's College in 1986 for a history of the suburb of North Oxford which will be published by Yale University Press in 1992. I wish to thank the President and fellows for their support during three and a half years' work and for free access to the muniments of the College.

2   *Report of the Commissioners Appointed to Inquire into the Property and Income of the Universities of Oxford and Cambridge*, III, 1874.

3   C. M. Clode, *The Early History of the Guild of Merchant Taylors*, I, London, 1888, pp. 108 ff.

4   W. H. Stevenson and H. E. Salter, *The Early History of St John's College, Oxford*, Oxford, 1939, pp. 151 – 5.

5   Christopher Hill, *Economic Problems of the Church*, Oxford, 1956, p. 30.

6   R. J. Morris, 'The friars and paradise: an essay in the building history of Oxford, 1801 – 1861', *Oxoniensia*, XXXVI, 1971, pp. 72 – 98.

7   Morris, 'The friars', p. 72.

8   Christopher Brooke and Roger Highfield, *Oxford and Cambridge*, Cambridge, 1988, pp. 171 – 2.

9   St John's College (SJC), *Register*, 24 October 1804.

10   SJC, *Register*, 8 April 1809, 3 April 1811.

11   SJC, *Register*, 9 October 1822.

12   *Jackson's Oxford Journal* (*JOJ*), 12 April 1823.

13   SJC, *Register*, 8 October 1823.

14   SJC, Muniments EST III, MP 185.

15   Anson Osmond, 'Building on the Beaumonts: an example of early 19th-century housing development', *Oxoniensia*, XLIX, 1984, pp. 301 – 25.

16   SJC, *Register*, 6 April 1825; *JOJ*, 20 October 1827.

17   10 Geo IV, c. 15.

18   SJC, Muniments VB 91.

19   SJC, Muniments VB 101.

20   SJC, *Register*, 5 October 1842.

21   Oxford Country Record Office, PD2 57, 60.

22   *JOJ*, 8 September 1860; SJC, *The Bursar's Letters*, 1 December 1882.

23   SJC, *Register*, 10 April 1844, 30 January 1846.

24   *JOJ*, 3 March 1849.

25   SJC, Muniments VB 114.

26   *JOJ*, 19 March 1853. For Seckham see Peter Howell, 'Samuel Lipscomb Seckham', *Oxoniensia*, XLI, 1976, pp. 337 – 47.

27   Bodleian (Bodl.) MS Dep c. 541 item d. See Howell, above, p. 000.

28   Bodl., MS Dep b. 217.

29   SJC, *Register*, 7 October 1840.

30   SJC, Muniments EST III, MP 183.

31   SJC, *Register*, 13 October 1854; 18 and 19 Vict c. 10.

32   SJC, *General Ledger, 1841 – 1860*, p. 358.

33   *JOJ*, 5 April 1851.

34   Bodl., GA Oxon c. 152.

35   SJC, *Register*, 17 October 1862.

36   SJC, *Register*, 18 October 1867.

37   SJC, *Register*, 15 October 1859; Muniments VC 7, 8.

38 SJC, *Bursar's Incoming Letters*, 7 May 1879.

39 For Wilkinson see Andrew Saint, 'Three Oxford architects', *Oxoniensia*, XXXV, 1970, pp. 53 – 102.

40 SJC, Printed Building Agreements, Muniments V.

41 SJC, *Long Lease Books*.

42 SJC, *Register*, 14 October 1864. See also Howe, above, pp. 15ff.

43 *Census Returns*, 1871, RG 10 1439; *London Directory*, 1860.

44 SJC, Printed Building Agreements, Muniments V.

45 SJC, *College Leases*, Muniments V.

46 *JOJ*, 7 October 1876.

47 Bodl., GA Oxon c. 152.

48 *Oxford Chronicle*, 17 March 1883.

49 SJC, *Estates Committee*, 18 October 1880.

50 For the effect of the agricultural depression on the finances of the colleges see J. P. D. Dunbabin, 'Oxford and Cambridge colleges finances, 1871 – 1913', *Economic History Review*, XXVIII, 1975, pp. 631 – 47, XXXI, 1978, pp. 446 – 9; A. J. Engel, 'Oxford college finances, 1871 – 1913: a comment', *Economic History Review*, XXXI, 1978, pp. 437 – 45.

51 *Report of the Commissioners*, I, 1874.

52 SJC, *Bursar's Letters*, 17 November 1883.

53 SJC, *Long Leases*.

54 SJC, *Bursar's Letters*, 17 November 1883.

55 SJC, *Estates Committee*, 6 February 1885.

56 SJC, *Estates Committee*, 26 February 1886.

57 40 and 41 Vict c. 48.

58 Brooke and Highfield, *Oxford and Cambridge*, p. 277.

59 R. C. Whiting, 'The university and its locality', in B. Harrison (ed.), *History of the University of Oxford*, VIII, Oxford, forthcoming.

60 SJC, *Register*, 31 January 1913.

61 SJC, *Estates Committee*, 7 February 1934. On the Science area, see Howell, above, p. 79.

62 SJC, *Register*, 24 June 1920.

63 SJC, *Register*, 20 January 1948.

64 SJC, *Register*, 4 February 1950.

65 SJC, Muniments Box File A 25a.

66 SJC, Muniments Box File A 26c.

67 SJC, *Estates Committee*, 21 June 1960.

68 SJC, *Estates Committee Memoranda*, 9 January 1960.

69 SJC, Muniments ADMIN XVI.

70 15 – 16 Elizabeth II c. 88; SJC, Muniments Box File A 25n.

71 David Cannadine, *Lords and Landlords*, Leicester, 1983.

72 Donald J. Olsen, *Town Planning in London*, New Haven, CT, 1982, p. xx.

73 Letter from E. S. Dobbs to Arthur Garrard, 17 February 1961, *Estates Committee Memoranda*, 1961.

Responses to growth in modern Oxford

During the course of the nineteenth century, Oxford fell from 33rd to 68th in the list of English towns and cities ranked by size of population. With fewer than 50,000 permanent residents in 1901, life was still dominated by the University and the college fellows were content that this should be so. Indeed they had contributed to the slowness of change. They had delayed the arrival of the railway for some seven years in the 1840s, defeated the Great Western Railway's plan to build workshops in the 1860s and were engaged at the turn of the century in preventing the electrification of the tramways. All of this was justified on aesthetic and moral grounds.

The slowness of population growth had its counterpart in the limited expansion of the built-up area beyond the confines of the medieval walled city. Significantly the most extensive growth had been northwards, along the Banbury and Woodstock Roads, prompted at least in part by the statute of 1877 which allowed the college fellows to retain their fellowships when they married. The villas of Norham Gardens and beyond form the core of the present Victorian Suburb Conservation Area.[1] Elsewhere there was limited suburban development, most of it confined to the western fringes of the city close to the gasworks (1818), the Walton Street buildings of the University Press (1830) and the railway stations (1852). If the dons noticed these changes at all, their attitude was probably that of William Warde Fowler, classics tutor at Lincoln College and a keen walker and birdwatcher, who attributed the tranquillity of Oxford to the control over the town exercised by the University, observing that 'the only adverse element even at the present day is the gradual but steady expansion of building to the north, south and west'.[2]

Fowler also attributed the colonisation of Boars Hill to the adoption of the bicycle, and he was no doubt aware of the shop at No. 48 High Street where a young William Morris had a cycle-repair business. Later he might have noted with interest the new building around the corner in Longwall Street which Morris had erected in 1910 for the growing car-hire trade but, like most of his contemporaries, would have failed to appreciate the significance of the prototype Morris Oxford (Bullnose) car which Morris assembled here in 1912. There was no space in Longwall for the production of cars and Morris moved in that year to the old military college in Cowley, only two miles east of Magdalen Bridge, but a world away from the university city centred on Carfax. Little interest was taken in the Cowley factory which, in any case, was soon turned over to munitions work. The impact of Morris was rather seen in his introduction of the first motor bus to Oxford's streets in 1913, a welcome competitor to the ancient horse-drawn trams which by now had become a laughing-stock but which endured up to the First World War as a symbol of the old Oxford.

The transformation of Oxford began in 1920. In that year Morris Motors produced fewer than 2,000 cars but five years later, in 1925, the total exceeded 55,000. Success was entirely due to Morris's own mechanical and business skills, his adoption of assembly methods and his foresight in reducing the price of the popular Oxford model which had cost £590 in 1921 but only £260 in 1925. Further growth followed the establishment of the Pressed Steel Company on an adjacent site in 1926 and the adoption soon afterwards of the moving assembly line. The total workforce in the Oxford car industry, some 200 in 1919, had grown to 5,000 in 1925 and to 10,000 by the early 1930s, old coach-building skills giving way in the course of this decade to new metalworking ones.[3] Some of this labour was recruited locally as the younger college servants discovered an alternative to the low pay of university work, but large numbers were drawn from outside the city. Some travelled daily from surrounding towns and villages, from as far afield as Swindon and Reading, but Oxford was also a magnet to the unemployed of Wales and northern England.

Between 1921 and 1937 the population of Oxford, within the area covered by the boundary extension of 1929, grew from 67,290 to an estimated 96,350. No one could be unaware of the changes that were taking place. The implications of rapid population growth for the social, economic, and administrative development of Oxford and its immediate neighbourhood was the subject of a two-volume study carried out in the late 1930s for Barnett House, the Social Studies Department of the University.[4] This wide-ranging investigation, covering employment, housing, local government, planning, education, health, and other services – equivalent locally to the Barlow Report at the national scale – provides the foundation of those academic analyses of Oxford's development that have taken place over the course of the succeeding half-century.

Gilbert, a geographer, observed that the rate of Oxford's population growth between 1921 and 1931, + 19.7 per cent, was greater than that of any other conurbation in Great Britain with the exception of Bournemouth (including Poole and Christchurch) and Watford. Most of the increase was attributable to in-migration such that, by 1931, almost 44 per cent of the total population had been born outside the City or County of Oxfordshire.[5] Even allowing for the undergraduates – the 1931 Census was taken in Full Term – this was a very high proportion. Through the 1920s the city council struggled to provide housing for the newcomers, taking advantage of the subsidies afforded by successive Housing Acts to build new dwellings, most of them for renting but some also for sale. Demand nevertheless greatly exceeded supply, not helped by the generally depressed state of the private sector. After 1930, however, the situation changed as the council's attention shifted to slum clearance under the 1930 Act and as private builders finally began to respond to the need for new homes. Twelve hundred new houses were built in 1934 alone, more than double the number completed by private builders throughout the whole of the 1920s.[6] The total number of new houses built in Oxford between 1919 and 1937 was 7,177, two-thirds of them by private enterprise.

Social division

The social impact on Oxford of the new population was enormous, comparable at a different scale with that which took place in Banbury following the arrival of Alcan in the early 1930s.[7] A single statistic is revealing. In 1921 there were no fried-fish shops in Oxford; by 1935 there were eighteen of them, the largest concentration being in East Ward, where a high proportion of the newcomers had settled in close proximity to the motor works.[8] With East Oxford no doubt in mind, a contributor to the *Architectural Review* of 1929 commented: 'It would be ridiculous for those who have eyes to pretend that Oxford as a town today is greatly superior to Croydon or Burslem'.[9]

The occupational structure of the population had changed in the inter-war years. In 1920 the male workforce was largely made up of craftsmen and unskilled labourers, but the growth of the vehicle industry introduced a new group of semi-skilled workers, capable of earning as much as the traditional craftsmen.[10] But still more striking was the geographical separation of the different social classes, brought about by the polarisation of the housing market into public and private sectors, as well as by the actual distance that separated the car factories from the old centre of employment around the university. Speculative builders erected houses in an architectural style intended to distinguish their owners from council tenants, leading Emden and others to observe: 'The juxtaposition of clearly distinguishable private enterprise and council houses has also had unfortunate social effects. A cleavage is being established between the two groups of tenants which was almost unknown when they jostled each other in the same street in the centre of the town.'[11]

The nature and extent of these social divisions were demonstrated after the war in a number of investigations carried out by the sociologists Mogey and Collison. Chronologically the first of these was Mogey's (1956) comparative study of St Ebbe's and Barton. The former, a densely packed area of narrow streets to the south-west of the city centre, had been largely built up between 1820 and 1870 and was earmarked by the council for comprehensive redevelopment under the slum clearance legislation. Much of the housing was decayed, lacking the usual amenities, but there were many small shops, pubs, pawnbrokers and other small traders, with a strong sense of community and neighbourhood. Barton, by contrast, represented the new Oxford, a response to the demands created by the growth of the vehicle industry.

This estate, of just over a thousand houses, had been begun in 1937 to house 'slum' families from nearby Old Headington and Headington Quarry, but it was principally developed after 1946. Cut off from the rest of the city by the Northern Bypass, it was built on a north-facing slope that was unattractive to the private sector. Some of the houses were of traditional materials but many were erected from prefabricated and other kinds of factory-made units, and although two schools had been built there was not a single shop on the estate in the early 1950s. Like St Ebbe's, the population of Barton was mainly working-class, but in other respects the contrast could not have been greater. 'The absence of any commonly accepted set of standards of belief and action distinguishes Barton from the community of St Ebbe's. It is in fact not a localized society nor do its inhabitants feel loyal to an isolating set of social customs.'[12]

In the late 1950s Mogey and Collison looked at the class cleavages that had been created in Oxford as a whole by the influx of inter-war migrants.[13] For this purpose they made use of small area occupational data from the 1951 Census, Oxford being one of the first British cities to be investigated in this way. They divided the city into five radial sectors, making use of the river valleys and other open spaces which serve as buffers between the principal built-up areas, and each of these sectors was in turn divided concentrically by drawing circles at 1-, 2-, and 3-mile radii from the city centre. This permitted analysis, both by sector and by distance from Carfax, of the data which they aggregated into five social classes. Indices of segregation and of dissimilarity, measures respectively of the percentage of each area's population which would have to move to replicate the distribution of the entire population and of each of the other social classes, were used as measures of the geographical separation of the five different social groups.

Amongst the conclusions to emerge from this study was the high degree of separation of Social Class I with an index of segregation of 35, the greatest measures of separation being, not unexpectedly, from Social Class V (index of dissimilarity of 46). Social Class II, which includes university and college teachers, was somewhat less segregated but still exhibited a much larger index of segregation (25) than the remaining three classes, Collison and Mogey attributing this to the effect of municipal housing.

In terms of geographical distribution, there was a heavy concentration of Social Classes I and II in the northern sector of the city, 40 per cent of this sector's adult population falling into these categories, double the percentage for Oxford as a whole. The innermost parts of this northern sector displayed particularly high concentrations of Social Classes I and II, Collison and Mogey contrasting Oxford in this respect with the typical American city, with its tendency for social class to rise towards the periphery. In Oxford, Social Class III (skilled occupations) was disproportionately represented towards the edge of the city, especially in the south-eastern sector, explicable in terms of the location of the vehicle industry and of municipal housing. A further consequence of the strong influence of car-making at Cowley was the higher index of segregation for Social Class III (13)

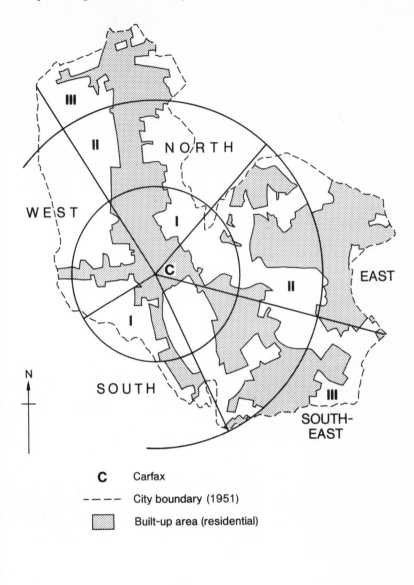

9 Collison and Mogey's social division of Oxford. From *American Journal of Sociology*, 1959, reproduced by permission of The University of Chicago Press

than for Class IV (8) in contrast with the observed pattern for most cities, where the index of segregation follows a U-shaped curve. There was, however, a concentration of the less skilled personal service group in the southern sector, including the not yet cleared St Ebbe's, where many college servants lived.[14]

The findings of Collison and Mogey relating to social segregation were broadly confirmed by Winchester, who utilised similar small area data from the 1961 Census and the Sample Census of 1966.[15] Social Class I remained as highly segregated as in the early 1950s but the index of segregation of Social Class II, which includes the academics, had fallen to 12 by 1961. This Winchester attributed to the growth and widening of the educational functions of Oxford, lecturers of various categories residing in many parts of the city. Social Class III, however, continued to display a greater than expected degree of segregation, evidence of the continuing social divide between the old city and that part of Oxford east of the Cherwell, where employment was dominated by the vehicle industry.

Indices of segregation and dissimilarity, even when based on data derived from small census enumeration districts, provide only a general indication of the geographical separation of the social classes, and the crudeness of these measures may obscure interesting local contrasts. This is evident in North Oxford, which is distinguished in all the studies as an area of high social status, but which includes a number of social barriers that are highly significant in behavioural terms. Gilbert drew attention to the 200-foot contour as a social dividing line in North Oxford.[16] It corresponds roughly with the edge of the gravel terrace on which the villas of Oxford's Victorian and Edwardian gentry were built. Below it, on the patches of lower terrace and on the river alluvium, were the dwellings of the poorer classes in quarters like that of Jericho, districts which had experienced the worst ravages of cholera and typhoid in the first half of the nineteenth century. Nowadays Jericho is a 'General Improvement Area' and has been 'gentrified', but until quite recently Walton Street and Kingston Road, which roughly follow the 200-foot contour, were proof of Gilbert's generalisation.[17]

Still more striking evidence of the force of social division is provided by the well-known saga of the Cutteslowe Walls.[18] Built across two roads in north Oxford in the early 1930s, the walls separated a private housing estate from an adjoining council estate and it was not until 1959 that the local authority obtained powers to demolish them.

Returning to the macro-scale, the broad social divisions within Oxford persist. It may no longer be the case that the bus conductors on the Banbury Road route are given periodic 'rests' on the Cowley run to enable them to recover from the verbal hectoring of North Oxford residents, but the latter retain considerable authority and influence.[19] Simmie and Hale have demonstrated this, for example, in terms of control over land use.[20] They examined the outcome of planning decisions in three wards of the city for the period 1953–73 and were able to show that land and property owners in North Ward achieved greater success in their planning applications than the corresponding owners in wards of lower social status. This the authors account for in terms of the degrees of power exercised by contending groups, some being in a better position to manipulate the planning system to their advantage than others. The latter theme was taken up at greater length in Simmie's *Power, Property and Corporation* London, (1981), which looks at the history of a number of major planning decisions taken in Oxford.

The urban economy

Expansion of the motor industry between the wars turned Oxford into a boom town, but as Gilbert pointed out, manufacturing was only one of four main functions performed by the city.[21] In order of historical development these other roles were those of a trading adn market town, seat of a university, and goal of tourists. To some extent the different activities could be seen as complementary, but in other respects they were in competition, not least for certain types of labour, as well as for housing and other services in a city whre space was at a premium. It is scarcely surprising, therefore, that the relationship of these functions to each other and their respective contributions to the urban economy should have become another theme judged worthy of academic analysis.

Oxford's dependence on the vehicle industry was recognised as early as the 1930s and has been a recurrent theme in studies of local employment structure ever since. By 1936 the car firms – Pressed Steel, Morris Motors, and the Radiators factory in the Woodstock Road – were employing between 10,000 and 11,000 workers, some 30 per cent of the insured workers in the Oxford area.[22] Other principal sources of male employment were the building trade, printing and publishing (the University Press with between 800 and 900 employees accounting for half the total), the smaller engineering firms of Lucy's and John Allen, and a number of craft industries, including boat-building. About a hundred women worked at Cooper's marmalade factory near the railway station, but most female employment was in domestic service or in jobs related to the university, landladies, for example. Because of the size of this service sector the ratio of occupied women to men, 49/100, was higher than the national average of 42.[23] The 1,100 servants employed by the colleges in 1936 were at that time mainly male.[24]

The range of work available in Oxford between the wars ensured a low rate of unemployment, even at the worst point of the depression in the early 1930s. The problem most commonly stressed was the tendency of the vehicle industry to sudden short spells of unemployment, in part due to irregularity in the supply of parts, in part to fluctuations in demand which included slack periods before the launch of a new model. Up to a quarter of the entire workforce could be laid off in a bad month.[25] Such fluctuations had implications for house purchase and contributed to the concern which began to mount in the 1930s about reliance on car manufacture and the need at some future date to encourage the provision of alternative sources of employment.

By 1946 the number employed in the Oxford motor industry exceeded 15,000.[26] In that same year the city council received letters from the Nuffield Organization and Pressed Steel about the provision of housing for the anticipated expansion of the two companies. Alarmed at the prospect of housing families of an additional 4,000 workers, the council arranged a conference with representatives of the two firms and the University. The Minister of Town and Country Planning, Lewis Silkin, was present at this meeting and he expressed the view, which the Council endorsed, 'that all possible steps be taken in an endeavour to prevent the population for which Oxford is the natural centre for increasing'. In response the Nuffield Organization declared that it could manage with its present workforce whilst Pressed Steel reduced its demands to an extra 2,000 employees.

The possibility of actually removing the motor works from Oxford altogether was a matter of quite serious debate in the 1940s. The most powerful advocate of the idea was Thomas Sharp, who, in *Oxford Replanned* (1948), described the city's dependence on the motor industry as 'unhealthy'. It was discussed at the meeting of the city council with representatives of the firms concerned in 1946 but the obvious difficulties were recognised on both sides and the idea was finally rejected in the City Development Plan of 1953.[27] A policy of restraint on growth was, however, incorporated in the Plan.

Despite the agreement to limit numbers to around 16,000, employment in the Oxford car industry continued to grow. Houston estimated a total of around 17,000 in the early 1950s, but expansion was rapid with the formation of the British Motor Corporation in 1952 and the growth in demand for vehicles nationally.[28] A peak of 26,860 was reached in 1963. This represented almost exactly one-third of total employment in the city at that time.

The failure of the City's no-growth policy to check the expansion in employment was noted by Gottmann, who observed that the 34.6 per cent increase in the size of Oxford's labour force between 1952 and 1968 was the highest in England and Wales.[29] The total number of jobs, about 75,000 in 1974, was out of all proportion to the size of the resident population of the city, then around 110,000, implying a considerable amount of commuting with all its strains on the local road network and transport services. The history of the 1930s seemed to have been repeated in the 1960s. The vehicle industry still accounted for approximately a third of all jobs in 1974.

The motor industry's dominance of the manufacturing sector of Oxford's economy was paralleled in the 1970s by the University's role in the service sector, to the extent that Gottmann was able to describe the city's workforce as 'bipolarized'.[30] The University and its colleges employed some 8,000 directly but to these, Gottmann suggested, should be added the still larger number employed in other educational establishments, in publishing and bookselling, and in the city's hospitals, most of which had links of various kinds with the University. He thus arrived at a total of 20,000 university-related jobs, to which the economic effect of some 11,000 students could be added in order to gauge the true significance of the University's influence on the city.

Gottmann uses the phrase 'interweaving of quaternary activites' to describe the linkage patterns that exist between a body such as the University and the many other institutions, trades, and activities that are, to a greater or lesser extent, dependent upon it. The nature of these links, involving the exchange of services and of information as well as of goods, was demonstrated by Baird in her account of a questionnaire and interview survey undertaken by the University School of Geography in the early 1970s: 'Many interviewees indicated

that the University or its members represented a significant part
of their market.'[31] The chain of linkages stemming from the University also extends to the hotels, guest houses, and specialist services
which cater for the needs of tourists visiting Oxford. Visitor numbers
are notoriously difficult to assess; so is their economic effect, but
of the impact of tourism on Oxford there can be little doubt. More
overseas visitors came to Oxford in the early 1970s than to any other
city apart from London, and recent years have seen a big growth in
the conference trade, of particular advantage to the colleges.[32]

The rapid expansion which characterised the vehicle industry in the
1960s and early 1970s has been reversed over the last decade or so.
Competition for markets has led to rationalisation and the replacement
of assembly workers by robots so that, by 1988, the number of car
workers in Oxford had fallen to around 10,500, similar to the total
recorded half a century earlier. Closure of the North and South Works
in the early 1990s will further reduce that number. The high unemployment figures of the early 1980s gave rise to renewed concern about
Oxford's dependence on a narrow manufacturing base and to calls for
encouragement to be given to the search for alternative forms of employment. Such recruitment would seem unnecessary, however. Oxford's
central position in southern England made it attractive to firms moving
from congested sites in London, Birmingham, and elsewhere, a
tendency noted as long ago as the 1960s, whilst the University's
laboratories are increasingly involved in the generation locally of
modern science-related industries.[33] The problem in the late 1980s
was therefore less one of creating jobs than of finding the space
for them to be located.

Roads and land use

The medieval walled city of Oxford, situated on the southernmost
tip of the gravel terrace referred to above, is surrounded except
on the north by the low-lying alluvial plains of the rivers Thames
and Cherwell. Every year these rivers flood, and when the flooding
is extensive the old city stands out as an island in a great lake.[34] For
centuries the population of Oxford was largely confined to the walled
area and suburban development, when it took place, was guided by
the presence of patches of low-lying gravel which afforded sites that
were reasonably safe from the flood hazard. The result has been to
impart a curious spider-like shape to the built-up area, tentacles of

building extending outwards from Carfax. To the east of Magdalen Bridge, where twentieth-century development has foundations in more solid rocks, the shape is more compact, though even here the built-up area is interrupted by wedges of open space like that of South Park and Southfield. The tentacular shape of Oxford reinforces the social divisions discussed above and, in addition, provides the clue to many of the city's planning problems, not least those to do with roads and traffic.

Most cities experience traffic congestion at the centre but in Oxford's case this is exaggerated by the emphasis on radial movement consequent upon the city's distinctive layout. Traffic converges on Carfax, the High Street and Magdalen Bridge, the only crossing of the Cherwell until modern times. Furthermore it is encouraged to do so by the geographical separation of land uses that has come about during the present century. In particular, the principal concentration of population in modern Oxford, east of the Cherwell, is separated by the university quarter from the main shops, administrative offices, and transport terminals that are centred on Cornmarket and the area to the west. As an American observer put it: 'Geographically the situation is as if residents of Leamington Spa had to journey to Warwick to purchase, or as if the housewives of St Paul could reach adequate stores only by going to Minneapolis.'[35] The problem has been made worse by what Ackroyd described as a 'high degree of car-mindedness'.[36] In 1937 Oxford possessed 95 motor vehicles per thousand of its population compared with an average for England Wales as a whole of only 66. The corresponding figures for private cars alone were 71 and 41. Then there are the cyclists. A traffic census carried out in 1938 discovered that over 19,200 bicycles a day crossed Magdalen Bridge, making this the point of highest concentration of cycle traffic in the country. The corresponding figure for motor vehicles was 16,760.

As a market town, Oxford draws in people from a wide rural area, providing shopping and higher-order services for a population at least three times the size of the city itself. It also lies at a crossroads in the centre of southern England and therefore attracts a good deal of through traffic in addition to the tourists who come to visit. A ring road was begun in the early 1930s but this was not completed until the mid-1960s, which meant that both long-distance and local traffic converged on Carfax. Chesterton described the Cornmarket of the 1950s as 'at the same time a shoppers' promenade and the principal north – south route through the centre of England'.[37] A traffic survey carried out in 1957 showed that little more than half the vehicles entering the city centre had the object of their journey there. Some 15 per cent was through traffic; another 30 per cent was inter-neighbourhood traffic compelled to use the centre because of the lack of bypasses and link roads.[38] Donnington Bridge, which links the Abingdon and Iffley Roads, was not opened until 1962, whilst the Marston Ferry link between Summertown and Headington had to wait until 1971. Both had been proposed as early as the 1920s and if built earlier might have spared Oxford the agony of the Christ Church Meadow controversy.

The arguments for and against new roads have fuelled academic debate for at least half a century. The problem was simple – how to relieve the High Street of the intense traffic pressure that had built up as a result of the convergence of vehicles on Carfax and Magdalen Bridge. The solution was more illusive and, as the *Manchester Guardian* observed: 'there must have been almost as many university road proposals as dons with half-an-hour to spare'. They were aired in the local and national press, in *The Oxford Magazine* (the dons' newspaper) and in *Oxford* (publication of the Oxford Society). When the British Association met in Oxford in 1954 the delegates were addressed by the Vice-Chancellor on the subject.[39] The arguments were not untouched by self-interest as different parties sought to promote or to protect Christ Church Meadow, the University Parks, St Giles or Norham Gardens.

The debate about roads and land use was initiated in the 1940s and this was the decade that produced the most imaginative suggestions, some of which may be looked back upon as lost opportunities.[40] Foremost amongst the latter was the 'twin city' concept, seen by its protagonists as an alternative to the road across, or close to, Christ Church Meadow.

The Barnett House Survey of 1938 – 40 was critical of the changes taking place in the centre of the city around Carfax where the arrival of multiple stores was producing buildings unrelated to their neighbours and to a loss of character in some of the main thoroughfares. Since the possibilities for commercial expansion were restricted here by the presence of the University and its colleges, it was felt that Oxford's needs would be best served by building an entirely new shopping and administrative centre to the east of Magdalen Bridge. The effect of such a scheme would be to reduce the amount of traffic using

Magdalen Bridge and the High Street so that the historic centre of the city could 'revert to a type of business dependent upon such custom as the University and north Oxford, supplemented by the tourist traffic, could give'.

These views were echoed in a report of a committee on planning and reconstruction that had been set up by the Oxford Preservation Trust.[41] A. B. Emden, Principal of St Edmund Hall, who had acted as Chairman of the Barnett House planning group, was a member of this committee which was chaired, in turn, by Viscount Samuel. The Trust's report referred to the area immediately east of Magdalen Bridge as 'the geographical centre of Oxford' and proposed that a new civic centre be built here at The Plain. The interests of the 50,000 inhabitants of east Oxford – 'a great new town' – were also to be served by the creation of an important shopping centre and the upgrading of Cowley railway station. The twin-city idea was endorsed in general terms the following year in a booklet published by the Town Planning Committee of the city council, its Chairman having served on the Samuel Committee.[42] The council and the Trust were at one on shopping and the need to improve Cowley station but the city team rejected the plan for a civic centre at The Plain. However, Thomas Rayson, a local architect, returned to the merits of this location as a site for new buildings to serve both city and county, 'a magnificent block of buildings that leaves no room for the doubt that Oxford is not only a University but a City'.[43] His civic centre included a Great Hall and two smaller halls for music and drama. In addition there was to be a new shopping and social centre near Cowley.

The twin-city plans of Emden, Samuel, and others had its opponents in Lawrence Dale and Thomas Sharp, who dismissed it as segregationist, isolationist and escapist.[44] According to Sharp, the notion of a self-contained city east of Magdalen Bridge 'ignored all the realities'; its effect would be to denude the historical centre of the city 'to give a fillip to an unsatisfactory suburb'. In retrospect the twin-city idea can be said to have failed because of the emphasis which it put on civic offices and the insufficient attention given to the size and location of the commercial element in any new development. When the city's Development Plan was published in 1953 it included details of a new shopping and commercial precinct at Cowley but the first stage of this project was not completed until 1965.[45] By this time the opportunity of shifting the retail centre of gravity of Oxford had been lost, the turning-point probably being the permission given on appeal to Woolworths by the Minister, Harold Macmillan, to build a huge new store on the site of the Clarendon Hotel in Cornmarket Street. This decision paved the way for similar schemes by the other multiples. Another factor was the uncertainty that was still felt in 1953 over the scale of the proposed new estate at Blackbird Leys on which work was to begin in 1957. Had this scheme been more advanced it might have been possible to make more ambitious plans for the Cowley Centre. As it was, the latter was too small, too late, and possibly not sufficiently central, to act as core to the new Oxford. Thus were Cornmarket Street and Queen Street destined to assume their present form, where the merits of pedestrianisation have been lost to the pressures of competing bus services and where the last vestiges of architectural elegance are swamped by nondescript house styles and commercial gimmickry.

The origin of the Meadow Road idea is usually attributed to the architect Lawrence Dale, who put forward the suggestion in a pamphlet, published under a pseudonym, in 1941 and then elaborated upon it in his book, *Towards a Plan for Oxford City*, in 1944. His road crossed the southern part of Christ Church Meadow, bridging the Cherwell just about the New Cut and running close to the north bank of the Thames. When Thomas Sharp published his book, *Oxford Replanned*, in 1948, the road, which he called Merton Mall, had been moved nearer to the High Street and ran parallel to the Broad Walk.

Sharp's plan for Oxford is the most scholarly analysis of the city's planning problems that has ever been published. He saw the necessity of limiting, even reversing, the growth of the city if its character were to be preserved, and this he sought to do principally by removal of the motor works.[46] This done, he saw no necessity to transfer the commercial and administrative heart of Oxford to the east of Magdalen Bridge. Instead, his plan involved a Haussmannian transformation of the area lying to the west of Cornmarket in order to accommodate an expanded shopping and office core. Sharp is important because he set himself the task of determining what kind of city Oxford should be, seeking to reverse the process of industrialisation in favour of a return to its market town and university functions. The visionary element, however, tended to get lost in the inevitable controversy arounsed by his advocacy of the Mall.

The history of the Oxford roads dispute is well known and has been described in some detail by Newman.[47] When it was at its most heated in the mid-1950s the Vice-Chancellor was in favour of a Meadow road, but the official university position was one of opposition to any road between the Thames in the south and Norham Gardens in the north, at least until the effect of bypasses and other proposed relief roads could be gauged.[48] A letter to *The Times*, signed by thirteen college heads, referred to the 'priceless heritage' of the Meadow and declared that 'The logic of those who would save the High by ruining the Meadow and the Parks is the shocking logic of the false mother who agreed that the baby should be cut in half.'[49] In the end the argument that carried most weight was the one that the Meadow Road would only duplicate the problem of the High Street or, if the latter were closed, shift the congestion a short distance away. It was, understandably enough, the view of Christ Church and also the one advanced by Colin Buchanan, who represented university interests at public inquiry.[50]

The threat to Christ Church Meadow receded after the Minister rejected the plan in 1965. Thereafter attention turned to the routes of alternative inner relief roads, none of which have actually been built. By the early 1970s there had been a shift in opinion away from road-building towards traffic management.[51] This is evident in the city council's *Balanced Transport Policy* of 1973, the basis of most of the planning for traffic that has gone on in the city since that date. Contemplating the cows in Christ Church Meadow or the cricketers in the Parks, one can feel grateful for the delays occasioned by academic debate.

Conservation

The beauty of Oxford and its surroundings has never been in doubt and it has been widely extolled in both prose and poetry. But beauty is easily marred and the need to conserve, even to enhance that beauty has long been a matter of academic interest and concern. A classic example is the attempt made to prevent the expansion, and then to effect the removal of the gasworks from St Ebbe's, a matter that was finally resolved in the House of Lords.

Early in the century concern began to be expressed at the loss of Oxford's legacy of domestic architecture, first to the expansion of the colleges, later to the spread of commercial and related functions consequent upon the growth of the city as a whole. The style of these old houses varies but the most typical, sometimes referred to as the 'Christminster' house, is of seventeenth-century date, possibly built of stone but more commonly of timber with lath and plaster filling, its façade colour-washed or stuccoed. It has three storeys, the upper one sometimes projecting. Bays and oriel windows are not uncommon, whilst the upper storey is typically gabled, with mullioned lights set in large dormers. Holywell Street offers the most complete set of examples, but even here the continuity of housing on the south side was broken by the erection of New College's Scott building (1872–96) and, on the north side, by the creation of Mansfield Road in the 1890s.

It was to check the further erosion of domestic buildings that the Oxford Architectural and Historical Society set up an Old Houses Committee in 1912. The report of this Committee, made up of F. E. Howard, H. E. Salter and C. M. Toynbee, was published in 1914, observing that 'Oxford was in former times rich in beautiful houses of many periods; unhappily one after another has been demolished and there now remain only a few here and there to remind us of the civic antiquity of the town and to show us what was the character of its domestic architecture'. The report contained photographs and notes on just fourteen of the most outstanding buildings, including the Golden Cross, 26–28 Cornmarket Street (Zac's Macs – now Laura Ashley), Kemp Hall, Bishop King's Place, Littlemore Hall (Alice's Shop), and several houses in Holywell Street.

The exercise was repeated by the Society's Old Houses Committee in 1936, those responsible this time being J. N. L. Myres, E. T. Long and P. S. Spokes. Their list, published in the first edition of *Oxoniensia* and by the Oxford Preservation Trust, was much longer, containing all the individual houses thought worthy of preservation. 'Fifty years ago the domestic architecture of Oxford must have been of outstanding beauty and variety, and much of it has already been destroyed piecemeal; it is hoped that this report may form the basis for an agreed policy among those who realise the value of what remains.' It was pioneering work, especially in view of the fact that the Ministry of Housing did not begin its official 'listing' of old properties until 1944.

The same Committee of 1936 also drew attention in its report to 'several streets in Oxford whose beauty depends upon the existence of groups of houses', houses which achieved their effect as groups and as 'examples of that harmonious variety' which is a feature of older English street architecture. The whole north side of Holywell was considered to form such a group; another was the little group of houses in High Street between Queen's and All Souls that includes Drawda Hall. This recognition given, both to the setting of individual buildings and to the importance of variety in the street scene, was equally pioneering. It was taken up by Thomas Sharp who, in *Oxford Replanned*, laid stress on the value of 'townscape' and of domestic buildings acting as 'foils' to the grandeur of adjoining college architecture. These were ideas that were late to bear fruit in the Civic Amenities Act of 1967 which permitted local authorities to designate Conservation Areas.

The beauty of Oxford derives not only from its buildings but also from its setting. The floodland that has shaped the built-up area also ensures that meadows penetrate to the heart of the city and the close proximity of town and country has been noted by many writers. It was the rustic qualities of Christ Church Meadow, where cows graze, that swayed many of the opponents of the road scheme. Equally renowned are the views of the city – Matthew Arnold's 'dreaming spires' – from the hills that flank Oxford to east and west: Shotover, Elsfield, Wytham, Boars Hill. These classic views achieve their effect because of the encircling meadows from which the old city and its towers appear to rise.

But meadows can be drained and hill slopes with views are attractive as house sites. The threat became only too evident in the inter-war years when population growth and increasing car ownership led to suburbanisation, as at Cumnor. A perceptive Betjeman caught the spirit of the times: 'What an approach to the city of learning .... Here the half-timbered villa holds its own boldly beside the bogus-modern, here the bay windows and stained glass front door survey the niggling rock garden and arid crazy paving .... The Scholar Gypsy must wash his bronzed face in birdbaths and sleep under the shade of stone toad stools is he is still to roam the slopes of Cumnor Hill.'[52] It was the desire to control this kind of sprawling development that led to the establishment of the Oxford Preservation Trust in 1927. The foundation of the Trust was largely due to the enterprise of H. A. L. Fisher, Warden of New College, and Sir Michael Sadler, Master of University College, and its members sought to preserve the classic views of the city by purchasing land at critical locations, as on Boars Hill and in the Cherwell Valley.

Since the Second World War the threat of urban sprawl has been reduced, firstly by the introduction of development control as a result of the Town and Country Planning Act and, secondly, by the designation of the Oxford Green Belt in the late 1950s. The latter extends outwards from the main built-up area for a distance of some five or six miles, taking in the hills that frame the city to west and east. There is a presumption against development in green belts but that does not prevent applications being made and the success of green belt policy depends on the commitment of the local authorities concerned, in this case the city of Oxford and the surrounding foru district councils that make up the post-1974 County of Oxfordshire.

A weakness in the case of the Oxford Green Belt is that its inner portion has never received formal government approval; it remains the Interim Green Belt, its inner boundary awaiting adjustment following the completion of local plans. This has made it vulnerable to developments of the kind that favour an urban fringe location, especially sites close to the ring road which runs for a good part of its fifteen-mile length through the Green Belt.[53] Nearly a dozen sites have been the subject of applications to build superstores, science parks, and sports complexes but at the time of writing permission for all of them had been withheld. New roadworks, particularly to the north of the city, increase the likelihood of success in the future, however. Indeed the area around Pear Tree between Oxford and Kidlington has been identified as a modern Carfax where the attractions to commerce and industry are as strong as they have been historically at the central crossroads of the old city. Much of the land on the fringe of Oxford is owned by institutions, notably by colleges of the University, some of which are anxious to sell it to developers in order to increase their endowment.[54] Future analysis of Oxford's development is likely to focus on this fringe area of the city and the interplay there of forces, economic, political and aesthetic, that will determine its form in the years to come.

Notes

1   The significance of local industry in the nineteenth century and the development of North Oxford are considered in more detail in the chapters by Howe and Hinchcliffe, respectively.

2   W. W. Fowler, *A Year with Birds*, Oxford, 1886, reproduced in Gordon Ottewell (ed.), *Warde Fowler's Countryside*, Gloucester, 1985, pp. 30–1.

3   Television History Workshop, *Making Cars: A History of Car Making by the People who Make the Cars*, London, 1985, p. 46.

4 A.F.C. Bourdillon (ed.), *A Survey of the Social Services in the Oxford District, I, Economics and Government of a Changing Area. II, Local Administration in a Changing Area (Survey)*, Oxford, 1938, 1940.

5 R.F. Bretherton, 'Population', in *Survey*, I, p. 27.

6 A.B. Emden *et al.*, 'Housing', in *Survey*, II, p. 353.

7 Margaret Stacey, *Tradition and Change. A Study of Banbury*, Oxford, 1960, pp. 51–2, 169–70.

8 E. Ackroyd, 'Transport', in *Survey*, II, pp. 403–23.

9 J. Morris, *The Oxford Book of Oxford*, Oxford, 1978, p. 356.

10 J. Marschak, 'Industrial immigration', in *Survey*, I, pp. 63–70.

11 Emden *et al.*, 'Housing', p. 353.

12 J.M. Mogey, *Family and Neighbourhood. Two Studies in Oxford*, Oxford, 1956, p. 156.

13 P. Collison and J.M. Mogey, 'Residence and social class in Oxford', *American Journal of Sociology*, LXIV, 1959, pp. 599–605.

14 P. Collison, 'Occupation, education and housing in an English city,' *American Journal of Sociology*, LXV, 1960, pp. 588–97.

15 S. Winchester, 'The segregation of social groups in Oxford', in D. Smith and D.I. Scargill (eds.), *Oxford and its Region*, Oxford, 1975, pp. 62–7. The topic of segregation is also tackled in Whiting's chapter, below.

16 E.W. Gilbert, 'Geography', in *Survey*, I, pp. 1–24.

17 A.G. Crosby, 'The experience of gradual renewal in the Jericho district of Oxford', School of Geography research paper 25, Oxford, 1980.

18 P. Collison, *The Cutteslowe Walls. A Study in Social Class*, London, 1963.

19 J.G. Sinclair, *Portrait of Oxford*, Sturry, 1931.

20 J.M. Simmie and D.J. Hale, 'The distributional effects of ownership and control of land use in Oxford', *Urban Studies*, XV, 1978, pp. 9–21.

21 E.W. Gilbert, 'The industrialization of Oxford', *The Geographical Journal*, CIX, 1947, pp. 1–25.

22 E. Ackroyd and A. Plummer, 'Industry', in *Survey*, I, pp. 71–98.

23 Marschak, 'Immigration', pp. 63–70.

24 Gilbert, 'Industrialization', pp. 1–25.

25 Gilbert, 'Industrialization', pp. 1–25.

26 City of Oxford, *City of Oxford Development Plan*, Oxford, 1953.

27 Oxford city council minutes, 1 July 1946.

28 J.M. Houston, 'Industries', in A.F. Martin and R.W. Steel (eds.), *The Oxford Region: A Scientific and Historical Survey*, Oxford, 1954, pp. 141–6.

29 J. Gottmann, 'The centrality of Oxford', in Smith and Scargill, *Oxford and its Region*, pp. 44–7.

30 Gottmann, 'The centrality'.

31 Barbara Baird, 'The interweaving of quaternary activities in Oxford', in Smith and Scargill, *Oxford and its region*, pp. 48–54.

32 I.M. Cosgrove, 'Tourism in Oxford', in D. Smith and D.I. Scargill (eds.), *Oxford and its Region*, Oxford, 1975, pp. 83 – 7. M.J. Breakell, 'Tourism in the Oxford region', in T. Rowley (ed.), *The Oxford Region*, Oxford, 1980, pp. 139 – 47.

33   D.I. Scargill, 'Metropolitan influences in the Oxford region', *Geography*, LXII, 1967, pp. 157 – 65.

34   E.W. Gilbert, 'The city of Oxford', in K. Clayton (ed.), *Guide to London Excursions*, London, 1964.

35   R. Newman, 'The future of Oxford', *The American Oxonian*, 1948, pp. 1 – 17.

36   Ackroyd, 'Transport', pp. 403 – 23.

37   E. Chesterton, 'The Oxford road problem', *The Geographical Magazine*, XXVIII, 1956, p. 507, citing the *Manchester Guardian*.

38   City of Oxford Development Plan Review, 1964.

39   A.H. Smith, 'The closing of Magdalen Bridge', *Selected Essays and Addresses*, based on articles in the *Oxford Mail*, 6 and 7 October 1955, Oxford, 1963, pp. 58 – 66.

40   R. Newman, 'Town planning in Oxford', *Oxford*, IX, pp. 59 – 72.

41   Viscount Samuel, *Oxford: Report of Committee on Town Planning and Reconstruction*, Part II, Oxford, 1942.

42   G. Montague Harris, *City of Oxford: Plans for the Future*, Oxford, 1943.

43   T. Rayson, *The King is in His Counting House: A Prospect of Oxford*, Oxford, 1946. On Rayson as an architect see Howell, above, p. 80.

44   T. Sharp, *Oxford Replanned*, London, 1948.

45   D. Thomas *et al.*, 'The Oxford case studies', in *Flexibility and Commitment in Planning*, Leiden, 1983, pp. 154 – 205.

46   See also Waller, below, p. 180.

47   R. Newman, *The Road and Christ Church Meadow: the Oxford Inner Relief Road Controversy 1923 – 74*, Minster Lovell, 1988.

48   A.H. Smith, *Addresses*. See also Hinchcliffe, above, p. 102.

49   *The Times*, 19 July 1955.

50   J. Lowe, 'Christ Church and Oxford roads', *Oxford*, XIV, 1956, pp. 13 – 16.

51   J.M. Bailey, 'The evolution of transport policy in Oxford', in T. Rowley (ed.), *The Oxford Region*, Oxford, 1980, pp. 97 – 123.

52   J. Betjeman, *An Oxford University Chest*, Oxford, 1938, p. 107.

53   D.I. Scargill, 'Conservation and the Oxford green belt', in Rowley, *Oxford Region*, pp. 125 – 38.

54   M. Boddington, *The Oxford Green Belt*, Rural Planning Services Publication No. 6, Ipsden, 1979.

Infant welfare in inter-war Oxford

A study of the personnel and the services connected with infant welfare in Oxford before the Second World War demonstrates the continuity of power amongst a social elite, and more particularly the power of the women amongst this social elite. Ideals of less eligibility and self-help, held strongly in Oxford and elsewhere before the turn of the century, continued to influence the shape of welfare provision. Resources made available to the poor were to be kept to a minimum, so as not to encourage dependency, and the poor were to help themselves.

After the First World War, Oxford was not a town of great poverty, but there were pockets of poor, run-down housing and needy occupants in the cramped courts between the colleges, as well as areas of insanitary conditions in St Ebbe's, Jericho, St Aldate's, behind the central colleges, and St Clement's.[1] Local affairs were dominated by university men, and the other professional elite of any cathedral town – the medical men, solicitors, and churchmen, with their wives and daughters, a few of whom were themselves members of the professions. The council was politically Liberal or Conservative at this time – at least, the members voted Liberal or Conservative in national elections, though they often ran for local office under personal rather than party auspices. An old university statute which gave a proportion of seats on the council to university members may have reinforced the Conservatism of the council; it certainly left less room for working-class or tradesmen's representation. In 1917 there were sixty-three councillors, nine of whom were elected by the University. There was only one woman councillor, Miss Merivale, amongst their number.[2] For Oxford's councillors during most of the inter-war period, the proper sphere of town government was public sanitation, paving, lighting, parks, and schools. The Board of Guardians dealt with the destitute in the workhouse and Poor Law school, and dispensed some out-relief, although this last was kept to a minimum in Oxford with the help of Alderman Phelps, Provost of Oriel, longtime chairman of the local Charity Organisation Society, and a member of the 1904–09 Poor Law Comission. Welfare work was regarded by councillors as the sphere of the voluntary organisations and charities; Oxford had a proliferation of voluntary societies, for destitute girls, for the feeble-minded, the Oxford Police Aided Society for the Clothing of Poor Children, the Free Dispensary, the voluntary hospitals, the Nursing Associations, and the Infant Welfare Association.[3]

Amongst all these voluntary organisations, those concerned with infant welfare and the health and well-being of mothers – poorer mothers – are of particular interest in this period. Maternal and child welfare had been a philanthropic focus since before the turn of the century. This focus, connected originally with the work of late Victorian lady visitors, was sharpened by national outcry at the poor health of working-class male recruits to the Boer War. The way this national concern about adolescent and adult health was channelled into voluntary and state activity to promote infant health is the subject of Anna Davin's essay, 'Imperialism and Motherhood'.[4] The manner in which Oxford's philanthropic elite responded to this national concern followed a pattern of philanthropic activity characteristic of towns and cities throughout Britain.[5]

Nationally, women dominated the maternal and child welfare groups – sanitary aid societies, health visiting associations, milk banks, societies for schools for mothers, infant welfare centres. The women's efforts were backed by only a sprinkling of medical men.[6] There were so many of these societies in the first thirty years of the century that it is unavoidable to wonder whether work in the societies was at least as important for the women volunteers and the medical professionals providing help as for those being helped.[7] Infant welfare must have seemed a perfect area of voluntary and council work, at a time when there was a tension for Liberal and Conservative women between their growing presence in the public sphere, and their political need to demonstrate that women's proper place was in the home. Oxford had a large number of such women, public-spirited university wives and daughters who wished to make a contribution to their local community not as experts, but as enthusiastic amateurs.

Whether national or local, statutory or philanthropic, maternal and child health and welfare work flourished in Britain during the first forty years of the century. During this period several important laws were passed to encourage infant and maternal health – the 1902 Midwives Act, the 1908 Notification of Births Act (permissive), the 1915 Notification of Births Act (statutory), the 1918 Maternity and Child Welfare Act, and the 1936 Midwives Act.[8] In consequence, local authorities had an increasingly complex duty to discharge in the sphere of infant welfare, an area also catered for by local philanthropic bodies. This might have been expected to lead to conflict or overlap between the statutory and voluntary bodies. In Oxford in particular, with a well-established group of women volunteers matched by an active council maternal and child welfare subcommittee, there might have been clashes. What emerges, however, is a history marked more by co-operation than conflict, where the volunteers helped mould Oxford's sparse public service for mothers and infants to a pattern which fitted their own beliefs.

Many of Oxford's Couny Borough councillors were also staunch voluntary committee members; they kept the rates paid by Oxford citizens as low as they could, as councillors, and simultaneously devoted their time, a modicum of their money, and especially their expertise to the voluntary associations which aimed to ease or improve the lives of the poor of the town. And there were still a great many poor in the town. Sparse services cannot be explained by lack of need, despite the dramatic changes William Morris and his car factory brought to Oxford, apparent from the mid-1920s onwards, which kept unemployment to a minimum and brought expansion and prosperity to the area.[9] Little was spent by the council on poor mothers and children – the average for the period 1919–39 spent on all public health services was 1.5 per cent of the council's total budget – and maternal and child welfare accounted for less than 5 per cent of public health expenditure. To give a rough comparison with a borough which had a similar population but a different attitude to welfare, in real figures Oxford contributed between £800 and £2,000 per annum to infant welfare during the 1920s, while Tottenham in the same period spent between £5,000 and £7,000.[10]

A record of Oxford in the 1920s contains plenty of references to hardship; families living in tents like the man who came to Croydon for work at the car factory, bringing his four children who had previously been confined to the workhouse. He arrived in Oxford only to find housing difficult to find and too expensive even on his relatively good salary of 80*s* a week, so with commendable ingenuity he put up a bell-tent for himself and his children, having calculated that the only way to keep his children warm and fed was to avoid rent. The National Society for the Prevention of Cruelty to Children, (NSPCC) had brought him to trial charged with negligence: the *Oxford Times* quotes the following part of his defence: 'in Oxford I find they are going to spend £5000 for housing wild animals, but they will not spend anything on housing human beings'.[11]

Other families suffering from the housing shortage were split up, like this one:

In one case a broken-hearted mother has had to part with three of her children, sent to the Cowley Road Workhouse, and has maintainence of 7/6d a week to pay for them, and if she cannot get accommodation for them in three weeks two of them will have to go to the Cowley Schools [the workhouse residential school]. Oxford City Council can act fast enough in making motor parks and garages; why don't they make a supply of proper houses for such families to live in? I think the City Council ought to wake up, and give this mother a house so that she and her husband can have the little ones with them.[12]

Statistics from the voluntary societies also give an indication of hardship; the Oxford Police Aided Association for the Clothing of Poor Children distributed 397 garments (all conspicuously marked and only lent, not given) and 70 pairs of boots in 1922. During 1937 and 1938 1,664 garments and 280 pairs of boots were distributed.[13] There seems little doubt of the existence of need in inter-war Oxford.

One of Oxford's foremost voluntary societies was the Infant Welfare Association, whose work started in 1905 as part of the responsibilities of the Sanitary Aid Association (SAA), itself begun in 1902 'for the purpose of improving sanitary and housing conditions and general health in Oxford'.[14] In 1905 they were known as the Health Committee of the SAA, set up to educate poor mothers in child-rearing in order to protect their infants from disease and death.[15] Some inner wards of Oxford had high infant mortality rates; the volunteer health visitors of this association claimed responsibility for a dramatic reduction in these rates by 1909, even after 'allowances for climatic conditions the Committee believe this decrease tends to prove that their work is really bearing fruit in an increase of knowledge of the laws of health among mothers.'[16]

The Association continued activities during the First World War, having become the Oxford Health and Housing Association in 1912. This amalgamation occurred because it was recognised at the time that housing and infant health were intimately linked: by 1921, however, public attitudes had changed, and the two functions were separated, one wing becoming the Infant Welfare Association (IWA). This association is interesting from several points of view. Its committee demonstrates a remarkable continuity of membership from 1905 to 1952 when the IWA finally disbanded. Brian Harrison has described these dominant women.[17] High on the list is Mrs Prichard, a surgeon's daughter with a first-class honours degree from Oxford. She was married to the Professor of Moral Philosophy, and had been one of the quartet of don's wives who set up the Sanitary Aid Society in 1902. She continued in this group until the end, following its many metamorphoses. Co-opted onto the Council subcommittee for Maternal and Child Welfare in 1919, she was chair from 1925 to 1931, and vice-chair from 1931 to 1937.[18] In 1919, Mrs Prichard stood unsuccessfully as a Conservative candidate for East Ward, on an infant welfare platform. She finally became a councillor in 1924 by standing for the University. Mrs Prichard was active in several other bodies in her long life of public service; the voluntary Association for the Feeble Minded, the Council Mental Deficiency Committee, the Council Education Committee, the Old Age Pension Committee, the Watch Committee, the post-1948 Children's Committee, and the NSPCC. As a young woman, enjoying the companionship of philanthropists Mrs A. Toynbee and Mrs T. H. Green, she had been influenced by the teachings of T. H. Green. Mrs Prichard had been a member of the Women's Co-operative Guild – Oxford's version was rather genteel, showing lantern slides of Italy to the respectable working class of Jericho – and a member of the local Christian Socialist Union, also rather more paternalistic than it appears to have been nationally.[19]

Mrs H. A. L. Fisher was also part of the founding Sanitary Aid Association, although by the inter-war period she had moved on to national prominence as a writer and campaigner on 'citizenship', and the founder of the association for 'the Unmarried Mother and her Child'. She retained her interest in the voluntary movement throughout: 'Fortunately in this country of ours, with its strong instinct for social organisation, its traditions of self-help, there is probably no great danger of limiting unduly the possibilities of the

voluntary workers. But there is some danger, however slight, and
it is well to remember it, and to understand and appreciate the
scope and the value of voluntary work.'[20]

Mrs Wells, married to the Warden of Wadham, and Mrs A. L.
Smith, married to the Master of Balliol, were the remaining members
of the original quartet. Both remained active in infant welfare into
the inter-war period. Mrs Wells, another first-class honours graduate
from Oxford, had been co-opted with Mrs Prichard to the Council
Maternal and Child Welfare Subcommittee in 1919, with Mrs Prichard.
These four powerful women embraced voluntary and statutory
responsibilities. Their circle included the publicly employed Dr
Ormerod, Medical Officer of Health, and L. R. Phelps. The IWA's
work, and the connection of this work with the city's growing public
health department through the 1920s and 1930s, is an example of
the changing relationship between voluntary and statutory agencies,
relating to services for mothers and children. In this case the voluntary
society's activities kept a check on the public health services. The
attitudes of the IWA committee, attitudes applauding self-help,
suspicious of the long term use of free material and medical help,
persisted, ensuring that although advice abounded milk, medical
treatment, convalescence, and nurseries had to be paid for by those
who used them.

There were twelve infant welfare centres operating in the County
Borough of Oxford in the 1920s, strategically placed to encourage
the less well-off to attend. The following quotation is a description
of one by the university wife who ran it, Mrs A. L. Smith: 'groups
of from forty to sixty (mothers) allow a real intimacy between the
helpers and the helped: problems are talked over, lifelong friendships
formed, sunshine brought into the lives of the plucky, struggling
mothers, and not less into other lives which, like my own, lacked
for many years such a sphere of usefulness'.[21]

On the surface this passage evokes a lively set of relationships
beween women of different social classes in inter-war Oxford. Closer
examination reveals some questions; what of mothers who lacked
'pluck'? (and what is pluck anyway?) What did Mrs Smith mean by
'sunshine' – for the helpers or the helped? How important to her,
or to the other Oxford helpers, was the 'sphere of usefulness' that
the clinics represented? Recent work by Hilary Marland on the
nationally acclaimed Huddersfield experiment suggests that the
tangible help for poor mothers and infants brought by the Mayor's

infant welfare initiative was negligible in comparison to the national acclaim this activity won for the Mayor, Mr B. Broadbent.[22]

Clinics for mothers and babies were a feature of life in most parts of Britain in the inter-war years. They were held in the poorer districts of many British towns and cities, and also in a number of villages. Some clinics, like the one run by Mrs Smith, were run by volunteers – always women, often (although not always) wives and daughters of professional men, highly educated and capable, but not in paid employment. Medical practitioners and nurses or health visitors, paid from a mixture of rates and national grants, ran clinics in other areas, or regularly attended local volunteer-run clinics. Physically, these clinics ranged from purpose-built premises equipped with weighing scales, examination couches, and consultation rooms, to draughty church halls hired for an hour once a month. Mothers who attended received advice on the various aspects of child-rearing, from feeding to clothing and how to manage difficult behaviour. They might be given the chance to buy recipes, magazines, wool, malt, dried or fresh milk, or a range of other goods at cost price. The doctor or health visitor would advise mothers to take children to their medical practitioner or the hospital outpatients on examination if there was anything wrong; it was not the clinic's role to provide treatment, merely to give guidance on the prevention of ill health.

What did Oxford's clinics offer? In 1905 the Sanitary Aid Association began a scheme of voluntary health visiting for all Oxford's notified newborn, and persuaded the councillors to provide a bottle of disinfectant to be given free to mothers on infant registration.[23] For a short time, Oxford ran a milk scheme, to provide cost price fresh milk to poor mothers, but this venture was abandoned and instead the committee concentrated on the following: a mother's thrift club, series of talks on child rearing, a comprehensive health visiting scheme for poorer mothers, a scheme for selling babies' bottles at cost price, a pram leasing scheme, and weekly or fortnightly baby weighing and advice clinics for mothers.[24] In 1919 there were seven of these clinics, and in 1939, thirteen. Gradually through this period the local council public health team – health visitors and medical practitioners/ medical officers – assumed greater prominence, and the volunteers and the Infant Welfare Association fell into a supporting role. Infant Welfare clinics became one of a range of 'official' services for mothers and infants provided in the late 1930s – ante-natal clinics, a maternity wing of the Radcliffe Infirmary (the local voluntary hospital), a nursery school, a hospital infant treatment clinic, along with the old 'voluntary' groups such as the NSPCC and the Oxford Police Aided Association for the Clothing of Poor Children.

July 1917 was a time of intense activity for infant welfare campaigners throughout Britain. National Baby Week had been arranged, instigated by the National Baby Week Council, to stimulate local efforts to reduce the number of infant deaths amongst British working-class families. A film was produced, which local groups could hire; a group of speakers were available on invitation, and local councils and voluntary groups invited to participate.[25] Oxford's voluntary association's (by now called the Oxford Health and Housing Association, or OHHA) response was to arrange a full programme of talks, processions, baby shows, demonstrations, open days at the infant welfare centres, and twice-nightly showings of the National Baby Week film, 'Mothercraft'. The stage management of the event was left to the Mrs Wells, Prichard, and Fisher, who formed the executive committee of the OHHA; they persuaded their President, the Regius Professor of Medicine, the celebrated Sir William Osler, to make the opening speech before the first showing of the film. Mrs Henry Irving, the well-known actress who starred as a health visitor in 'Mothercraft', came to Oxford to help with National Baby Week; her brother was the then Master of Balliol, A. L. Smith, whose wife was on the OHHA committee. These were powerful figures, in national as well as local spheres. According to reports in the *Oxford Journal* and the *Oxford Times*, National Baby Week was a huge success; the film played twice-nightly for five nights, to packed audiences, and judging from the pictures of local mothers and babies at teas on Balliol college steps and in Oriel College's gardens, Oxford's poorer mothers were prepared to take their part in the proceedings.[26]

The message given to Oxford citizens during this week was that they should produce more babies, to be reared to a new standard of excellence through the advisory work of the OHHA. There was also a recognition at this point in the First World War that rearing healthy babies also depended on the availability of good housing and good wages. Sir William Osler mentioned this in his speech, and the Oxford Citizen's Association – Mr Wells and Mr A. L. Smith were on the committee – campaigned for public housing and better public health in Oxford. This period of the war appears to be the only time until the late 1930s when Oxford's elite considered the importance of material well-being to infant health. Before and after this period, mothers and infants were seen as most in need of advice, not services or material goods. Volunteers could do much of this, but the OHHA committee recognised that some expert medical advice might be needed, and medical obstetric and paediatric skill ought to be available in the city: 'the city would do well to make the appointment of a lady as assistant Medical Officer of Health a permanent feature of its Health staff'.[27] Voluntary subscriptions would not be enough to pay these fees and wages, so state grants were applied for. The OHHA Annual Report of 1918–19 pressed for publicly-financed medical advice for mothers and infants – health visitors, general practitioner medical advisers, and a properly supervised maternity home – to augment the work of the volunteers.[28] Earlier, the OHHA had successfully campaigned for official health visitors to work with referrals from the volunteers, and an out-patient clinic for sick babies at the Radcliffe Infirmary. The Maternity and Child Welfare Act of 1918 made grants available to councils and voluntary organisations for a wide variety of facilities, from free meals and holidays through to health visitors and inspectors of midwives. Oxford, its council and its voluntary bodies continued to provide more advice than help. Six maternity beds were available in the Radcliffe Infirmary Maternity Home which opened in 1920, secured by a 50 per cent annual government grant of £500, but mothers paid for their confinements unless they proved hardship. A national Milk Order of 1919 allowed councils to provide free milk for mothers and infants; Oxford made milk available, but only after applicants had been assessed by the Medical Officer of Health, paid for the milk themselves, and claimed the money back from the Town Hall.[29]

The OHHA retained its influence over public maternal and child welfare in Oxford very simply. The Mother and Child Welfare Act decreed that a maternal and child welfare committee or sub-committee should be constituted in each local authority, or mother and child welfare affairs should be dealt with by an existing committee, and that these committees should contain at least two women, to be co-opted if necessary. Oxford's two women were Mrs Prichard and Mrs Wells. Oxford's provision remained limited. Infant welfare never regained the public prominence of the period between 1917 and 1920. Free provision was harshly means-tested in comparison with other authorities, and take-up was small, perhaps because of the process to which the applicant was subjected.[30] The major extensions of provision – the appointment of a maternal and child welfare

assistant medical officer in 1933, the employment of general practitioners in infant clinics for advice, the setting up of two ante-natal
clinics in 1932 and 1934, and the opening of a birth control clinic
for the very sick and very poor in the Radcliffe Infirmary in 1935,
were due in the first instance to Ministry of Health criticism, and
finally to the energy and determination of Dr Mary Fisher, the
Assistant Medical Officer of Health for maternity and child welfare
from 1934. Power slipped from the IWA under the Local Government
Act of 1929. This act meant that all voluntary bodies ceased to
make contracts and obtain grants from the Ministry of Health direct,
and instead obtained them through their local authority. The IWA
clinics were as a consequence taken over by Oxford County Borough
Council, and in 1936 the volunteers who ran the clinics were demoted
to volunteer helpers.[31]

Many infant welfare centres in Oxford retained an aura of church
visiting, something the rich did to the poor, left from the era of
T. H. Green. The following succinct and effective descriptions from
the Public Health Survey, carried out in 1931 by government inspectors
from the Ministry of Health, serve to illustrate this:

Nine welfare centres are run by the Oxford Infant Welfare Association,
and two taken over on the extension of the City boundaries, by the Council
direct. A grant of £57 is paid to the Voluntary Association.

One of the criticisms of the scheme has been that no doctor attended
these centres. This was remedied last year, and Dr Hill [the MOH] now
endeavours to attend as often as possible at ten of them. The eleventh,
held at Cowley Road Congregational School, is run by a Mrs A. L. Smith,
on the lines of a mothers meeting, and it is not considered worthwhile
sending either a doctor or a Health Visitor. It receives no share of the
grant. Health Visitors attend all the other centres. No treatment is given;
the babies are weighed, and dried milk, malt and oil, and baby clothes are
sold at cost price. Formerly short talks were given, but the meetings are
now too crowded and these have been abandoned.

Dr Hill tries to examine every new child, but his visits are necessarily
somewhat irregular. It is hoped that the appointment of a new Medical
Officer will make it possible to have a doctor always in attendance.

I visited several of the centres and although they were somewhat crowded,
the standard of accommodation and the facilities offered were up to standard.

Dr Williams asked me to visit particularly one at Alma Place, which he
hopes someday to close. Here some thirty or 40 children and their mothers
were crowded into a small upper room which could only be approached
by a narrow winding staircase. The room was lit by gas and had a distinct

smell of gas, in addition to being stuffy and overcrowded. Dr Hill, looking like a fortune teller, was trying to examine children in a corner of the room behind a green and red curtain. His accomodation here was in marked contrast to that at another clinic, where he examines children in the chancel of a church.[32]

Spiritual nurturing was in fact still part of the agenda for mothers' education, as it had been in the Mothers' Meetings of the nineteenth century.[33] Dr Mary Fisher still remembers with some amazement her interview for the medical officer's job in 1934, when Mrs Prichard, then Chair of the Maternal and Child Welfare subcommittee, asked for assurances that a concern for the spiritual welfare of Oxford mothers would take priority in her work.[34]

This description of a gradual increase in Oxford's helping agencies, and a gradual decrese in the power of voluntary bodies, superficially looks like a perfect example of the road to the British welfare state provision of the 1940s.[35] Looked at in more detail, it has been possible to discern another contradictory theme, that of the continuing presence of the powerful men and women of the voluntary agencies within the newer Oxford County Borough Council services, acting as a wet blanket over Oxford's free services, and limiting the scope of rate-borne provision at least until the 1940s. The same names appear on the executive committees of the IWA, the NSPCC, and the County Borough Maternity and Child Welfare Subcommittee; the same values that had driven the formation of the Sanitary Aid society in 1902 continue in the County Borough Council's Annual Reports of the 1930s.

Compared with state infant welfare facilities in other parts of Britain, facilities offered to mothers and children were few. By 1936 in Tottenham, for instance, a moderately wealthy greater London borough, mothers and infants could choose from a wide range of hospital and midwifery services, minor ailments clinics, and crèche facilities, in addition to post- and ante-natal clinics, and the ubiquitous mother's and infant's welfares. Tottenham's 1930s premises were for the most part modern and purpose-built, arranged in easy walking distance to all the borough's mothers, open many times a week; Oxford's draughty halls were in sorry contrast to this. Tottenham provided medical services, food, simple medicines, convalescent holidays, and crèche places free to families who passed a generous means test; Oxford's range of 'free' services extended only to milk (vitamins during the 1930s), outpatient infant consultation, and a very few confinements; Oxford's means tests were both stricter and more difficult to apply for than Tottenham's. Tottenham lacked an equivalent band of powerful conservative women volunteers. Occupants of the larger houses moved further into the country as London expanded, leaving Tottenham to be dominated by members of the Co-op party, members of the Nonconformist Brotherhood, who willingly put their weight behind good public health provision.[36]

What was the impact of Oxford's brand of maternal and child welfare on the lives of the people who were to be helped – the poor mothers and their infants? Deborah Dwork, in her book *War is Good For Babies*, advances the theory that the infant welfare centre, dispensing advice on modern motherhood, may have been a rather economical response to problems of high mortality and morbidity amongst infants, but was none the less successful. With this argument, Tottenham's Council could be accused of overkill, providing a more elaborate service than was strictly necessary in the interests of civic pride. To measure the success of Oxford's provision changes in infant mortality rates in Oxford between 1900 and 1940 follow, together with one mother's memories of pregnancy and childcare in the 1930s in Oxford.

Infant mortality rates in Oxford as a whole maintained a steady downward trend from the turn of the century, rather before the Sanitary Aid Association was formed. They began lower than the national average, and fell in parallel.[37] At the time, infant welfare activity was accepted as the cause of the fall, but with hindsight the causal link is not so certain. Only a certain proportion of women attended the clinics, and many attended only once or twice.[38] The mortality rates themselves, broken down by ward, show considerable fluctuation, even in areas with regularly large numbers of births. This is not to say that the clinics fulfilled no useful purpose; many women interviewed by Glyn Williams both enjoyed going to the clinics and were profoundly influenced by what they learnt.[39]

Another Oxford informant who went to the clinic 'once, but never again ... it was unhygienic ... the baby wet the seat ...', had rather a different view of infant welfare centres. She resented being checked up on 'by ... stuck-up volunteers'. She and her friend were keen on new motherhood methods, but they learnt these from magazines and the local chemist, not the clinics.[40] This distrust of public welfare is also echoed by one of the first Oxford health visitors, Miss Finucane, who remembers the hazards of giving advice: 'I must say they were inclined to breast feed ... but ... just when they thought they would .... That's what I had to get out of them, get them on the right road. Any old time would do, when they were crying. You had to be careful about weaning. You couldn't always rely on them to tell you the truth about it, to be quite honest.'[41]

The particular shape of infant welfare provision in Oxford was strongly influenced by a group of university wives who found in this work a 'sphere of usefulness' for themselves. The ethos pervading the public and the voluntary elements of this welfare work was a Liberal or Conservative one. Mothers should be advised and befriended, their spiritual welfare should be kept in mind, material help should be hard to obtain and only available in cases of illness and desperation. Bringing 'sunshine' into the lives of 'plucky' mothers cost nothing, but gave the appearance of a 'real' gift of health at a time when sunlight was seen as one of the most efficacious preventive health aids available. The infant welfare volunteers were an able group of women, who contributed a great deal to Oxford's civic life. But their response to the real material needs of mothers and children in Oxford was negligible, except in the brief period of post-war reconstruction between 1917 and 1920.

Notes

I am particularly grateful to Lara Marks and Charles Webster for their help at various stages in the production of this chapter.

1   A. F. C. Bourdillon (ed.), for the Barnett House Survey Committee, *A Survey of the Social Services in the Oxford District*, Oxford, vol. 1 1938; vol. 2 1940; Jessie Parfit, *The Health of a City: Oxford 1770–1974*, Oxford, 1987.

2   Oxford City Library (OCL), *County Borough Council Diary 1917–18*. For an explanation of the university role, see *The Oxford Magazine*, 25 May 1961, p. 371. See also Howe, above, p. 35, and Waller, p. 174.

3   *Oxford Times*, 1900–39, Annual Reports of voluntary societies.

4   Anna Davin, 'Imperialism and motherhood', *History Workshop Journal*, V, 1978, pp. 9–65; Anne Summers, 'A home from home – women's philanthropic work in the nineteenth century', in Sandra Burman (ed.), *Fit Work for Women*, London, 1979.

5   Jane Lewis, *The Politics of Motherhood*, London, 1980.

6   Lewis, *Politics of Motherhood*.

7   For another local example see Hilary Marland, 'A pioneer in infant welfare: the Huddersfield scheme', *Journal for the Social History of Medicine*, forthcoming.

8 For a summary of these acts, see John J. Clarke, *Outlines of Local Government of the United Kingdom*, Oxford, 1939, pp. 78, 82–3.

9 Bourdillon, *Survey*; R. C. Whiting, *The View from Cowley*, Oxford, 1983.

10 Oxford County Borough Council, *Treasurers' Reports*, 1919–39, annual tables on public health expenditure.

11 Oxford Times, 4 April 1930. The reference is to a new zoo in Kidlington, just north of Oxford.

12 *Oxford Times*, 12 November 1926, letters column.

13 Bodleian Library, *Annual Report*, Oxford Police Aided Society for the Clothing of Poor Children, 1937–38.

14 OCL, *Annual Report*, Sanitary Aid Association, 1908.

15 J. Stanton, 'Response to the Problem of Infant Mortality with Special Reference to the Infant Welfare Movement in Oxford 1902–18', University of London M.A. dissertation, 1979.

16 OCL, *Annual Report of the Sanitary Aid Association*, 1909.

17 Brian Harrison, 'Miss Butler's social survey', in A. H. Halsey (ed.), *Traditions of Social Policy*, Oxford 1976, pp. 27–72.

18 OCL, *Diaries* of Oxford County Borough Council, 1919–39.

19 Pusey House, Oxford, minute books, Women's Co-operative Guild, Co-op Hall, Christian Social Union.

20 Mrs H. A. L. Fisher, *The Citizen*, London, 1937, p. 198.

21 Mrs. A. L. Smith, *A Biography of A. L. Smith*, Oxford, 1928, p. 195.

22 Hilary Marland, 'Pioneer in infant werlfare'.

23 Stanton, 'Infant mortality'.

24 OCL, *Annual Report of the Sanitary Aid Association*, 1912.

25 See Jill Liddington, *The Life and Times of a Respectable Rebel*, London, 1984, pp. 266–8.

26 *Oxford Times*, 14 June 1917; *Oxford Journal*, 14 June 1917.

27 OCL, *Annual Report of the Oxford Health and Housing Committee*, 1918–19.

28 OCL, *Annual Report of the Oxford Health and Housing Committee*, 1918–19.

29 OCL, minute books, Maternal and Child Welfare Subcommittee of the Public Health Committee, Oxford County Borough Council, 1919–20.

30 See E. Peretz, 'Local studies in the building of a national maternity service 1920–40', in D. Foster and P. Swan (eds.), *Essays in Regional History*, Hull, 1992; 'The costs of modern motherhood to low income families in inter-war Britain', in V. Fildes (ed.), *Women and Children First. International Maternal and Infant Welfare 1800–1950*, London, forthcoming.

31 OCL, minute books, Maternal and Child Welfare Subcommittee, Oxford County Borough Council, 1936.

32 PRO, MH66/807, Public Health Survey.

33 Frank Prochaska, 'Body and soul: bible nurses and the poor in Victorian London', *Bulletin of the Institute of Historical Research*, IX, 143, 1987.

34 Interview with Dr Mary Fisher, Oxford, 1987.

35 For a more complex version of this transition see C. Webster, *The Health Services Since the War*, vol. I, London, 1988, chapter 1.

36 See. E. Peretz, 'A maternity service for England and Wales: local authority maternity care in the inter-war period in Oxfordshire and Tottenham', in J. Garcia *et al.* (eds.), *The Politics of Maternity Care*, Oxford, 1990.

37 D. Dwork, *War is Good for Babies and Other Young Children*, London, 1987.

38 F.J.G. Lishman, 'A survey of sixty years of infant mortality in a county borough, with special reference to preventability', *Public Health*, October 1937, pp. 13–22.

39 Glyn Williams, ' "Save the Babies" the infant welfare movement in Britain during the early twentieth century, with particular reference to the city of Oxford', unpublished ms, 1985.

40 Interview with Mrs Eldred, Oxford, 1985.

41 Interview with Miss Finucane, Oxford, 1985, quoted in 'The professionalisation of childcare', *Oral History Journal*, XVII, 1989, pp. 23–9.

Association and separation in the working class, 1920 – 1970

Oxford's working class in the twentieth century provides a fascinating example of coexistence and segregation in a community of contrasting occupations. In types of work experience it included the car workers at Cowley engaged in a mass-production industry, buffeted by a fluctuating market and embroiled in frequently acrimonious strikes, and the college servants, enjoying an equally distinctive experience but one more wholly associated with peace rather than disruption, and apparently insulated from the effects of rapid economic change. The car workers played a distinctive part in industrial relations from the 1920s to the 1970s, while the main characteristic of the college servants has been their very distance from the rhetoric and realities of 'the labour movement'. The two major economic interests in modern Oxford, the motor industry and the University, generated almost antithetical characteristics in their labour forces. In terms of scale, most other Oxford occupations were of course much nearer to the smaller institutions of the colleges than to the motor industry. As C. J. Day has commented, 'Beneath the car industry's lengthening shadows Oxford remained a city of small enterprises.'[1] Many of these fell into the service sector and were different in outlook and experience from workers employed in more recognisably industrial conditions. This sense of difference has been well caught by Alan Fox. Describing a London childhood, he has remembered the 'milkmen, dustmen, journeymen butchers and jobbing workshopmen (who) looked upon the organised working class as a class apart',[2] and much the same sort of dissimilarity has applied to Oxford. Some of the Oxford trades fell between these two categories: the printers, engineers, railwaymen, and skilled building workers had for the most part a background of union organisation and reasonably secure employment, and overall a much steadier existence than the car workers.

This kind of diversity is characteristic of many towns, but the interrelationships between the different groups have rarely been systematically studied. As the constraints upon industrial location diminished, the coexistence in the same town of large-scale factory employment and traditional trades became more rather than less common. The degrees of association and transfer between different occupations is an important question for urban and labour historians, and is the subject of this chapter. How far, in short, did Oxford's traditional working class maintain the characteristics of a small-town labour force, or was it susceptible to the influence of a major industry developing on the periphery at Cowley? This chapter addresses this question for the period from the 1920s to the 1970s, by which time the working class, and the districts in which they lived, had begun to be changed by the growth of technical and white-collar jobs associated with the expansion of the University.[3] The problem of the relationship of Cowley to Oxford is pursued first through aspects of geography, industrial relations, and social activity, and second through a study of recruitment to occupations and associations between them.

The peculiar geography of Oxford's urban development, which is fully explained in Ian Scargill's chapter in this volume, meant that Cowley expanded at some distance from the old town.[4] Even so, when the suburban growth took shape in the 1930s some felt that it was already too close to Oxford. The city engineer wrote in 1935: 'I remain unshaken in my belief that development of Oxford should be on higher land around the city, rather than on low lands within the city. The Horspath and Garsington hills are the ideal home for a goodly portion of the Oxford workers; and yet they are being packed in at 12 to an acre in lower Oxford.'[5]

Inevitably, Cowley developed as a strongly working-class area. Its housing, whether in the form of the privately-built estates of the 1930s or the later council provision of the 1950s and 1960s, was larger in scale and more uniform in character than anything in the older working-class districts. At Blackbird Leys, built in the later 1950s, it was decided against some opposition from the Conservatives not to allow any private housing on the estate. The high-rise blocks were unusual for Oxford but followed a pattern established

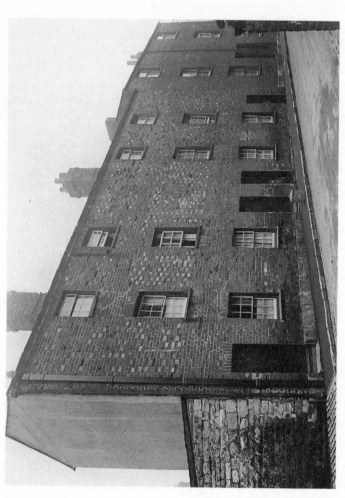

10 Caroline Street, East Oxford, in the 1930s. Shopkeepers and college servants, as well as unskilled labourers, lived in this street. *Oxfordshire Photographic Archive*

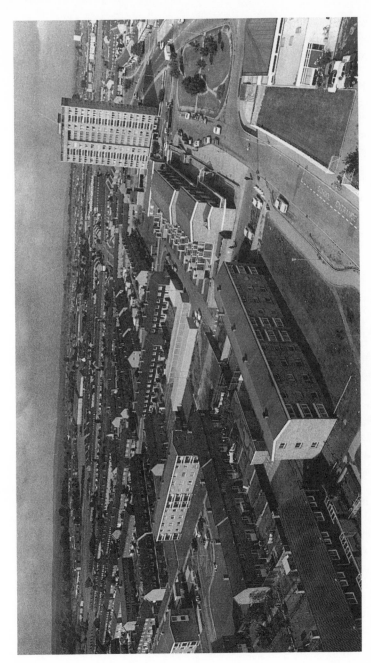

11 Blackbird Leys estate, begun in 1957. *Oxfordshire Photographic Archive*

elsewhere of encouraging vandalism and neglect. Blackbird Leys won a place alongside some London estates in Alice Coleman's seminal critique of these housing schemes in *Utopia on Trial*.

Styles of consumption were different, too. Many of the shops which developed in Cowley in the inter-war period were not branch extensions of those in the traditional town but separate entities.[6] Private enterprise, however, could not do enough to retain the Cowley shoppers in their own surroundings, and with municipal support a Cowley shopping centre was opened in 1962 which, not surprisingly, had a far higher proportion of working-class customers than the other Oxford shopping districts. Exclusion was never complete, for over 90 per cent of Cowley centre shoppers still also used those in the city centre, but it was judged in 1968 to have achieved some measure of success in keeping the Cowley population away from the old city.[7] The high earnings of the car workers had aroused resentment from the 1920s, and were reported even in times of adversity and low pay. When earnings were reduced by strikes in the 1970s a Cowley shop steward complained: 'Oxford people look down their noses at us car workers. They think we're muck, who earn more than we know how to spend, but they couldn't be more wrong.'[8] There may, however, have been some substance in the point that car workers did spend heavily from earnings when times were good. A survey of incomes and savings carried out in Oxford in 1951 found that the category into which car workers fell – semi-skilled machine minders – had a far lower level of liquid asset holding than the skilled workers (£98 as against £260), even though they earned more (£485 annually as against £444).[9] This survey occurred at a time of high spending on consumer durables which was consistent with a high level of dis-saving by car workers.

The sense of the Cowley works being geographically contiguous with Oxford but hardly part of it was enhanced rather than weakened by the industrial relations at the car factories. There were two aspects of this: one, organisations which might have acted as a bridge between the old and the new failed to do so; two, strikes at Cowley encouraged a particularly inward-looking perspective on the part of the workforce. In the early days it had looked as though the outcome might have been different. Trade union enthusiasts, who in the 1920s had struggled with diverse local groups amongst whom interest in the 'labour movement' was at best unevenly distributed, welcomed the new arrivals as an authentic, factory-based working class.[10] When the

Pressed Steel company was forced to recognise trade unions in 1934, this was the result of some vigorous local activity with Communist Party support, and some of this energy went into organising the busmen two years later. However, because the trades council, the local federation of trade unions, had a reputation for Communist sympathies, the national unions were wary of their local officials in Oxford becoming too closely involved in it. Additionally, the sheer numbers of car workers made any connections with longer-established local organisations extremely tenuous. Car workers had their own trade union branches at Cowley, and were not integrated into the much smaller ones to which the other Oxford workers belonged. As the motor industry grew in economic significance in the 1950s and trade unions were firmly established there, the Cowley shop stewards became more self-sufficient and had little sustained contact with organisations in the city.[11] Whereas in the 1930s the Cowley shop stewards had involved themselves in local strikes in other industries, by the 1950s this interest was less evident.[12]

The nature of strikes also worked in the same direction. The character of industrial relations in the motor industry over the whole of this period was shaped very much by specific conditions within each factory. General influences generated by the industry's economic performance inevitably made themselves felt, but the way the labour force was mobilised by its activists to press their claims encouraged a local and introspective mentality. The motor industry was characterised by volatility, in the degree of conflict as well as in variations between firms in the pattern of unionisation. Cowley showed both these characteristics to the full. The first company to set up there, Morris Motors, saw very little trade union development during the entire inter-war period, and no disputes worth recording. Union membership did develop in the favourable conditions of the Second World War but only became widespread after a large strike over redundancy in 1956.[13] This rather slow 'progress' contrasted sharply with the Pressed Steel factory next door which had been established in 1926 by an American firm. In an industry which experienced little by way of strikes and union growth in the inter-war years this factory saw the development of a major trade union base after 1934 for the Transport and General Workers' Union (T&GWU) and a rash of strikes. As these two firms were incorporated into a major car-producing conglomerate in the 1970s, Cowley none the less remained distinctive in its level of strikes. In 1983, for example, strikes at Cowley accounted for 24 per cent of the working days lost in the whole industry.[14]

What lay behind this history of turbulent industrial relations was the great leverage over the running of the factory which small groups of workers could exercise in the pursuit of higher earnings. Car factories consisted of a number of departments whose activities had to be interrelated and harmonised if production was to be efficient. From the 1920s pay was determined by piecework systems, and rates were struck for particular groups and departments. This focused most attention on the specific work group as a source of earnings and augmented the role of shop stewards in bargaining about pay. In the heyday of car workers' militancy in the 1960s, small groups had considerable power over total output and their shop stewards a major influence over trade union strategy in the factories. Indeed, one historian has argued that managements in the British motor industry consistently failed to exploit the opportunities provided by assembly line production for controlling the work regime, and therefore productivity, in the industry, largely because of the strength of labour resistance.[15] Many industrial problems are specific or parochial, but in the car factories they were unusually so. Workers in different departments contrasted strongly in their behaviour; a particular assembly line or paint shop might go through a turbulent spell and then become quieter. Whereas the Pressed Steel factory had been the source of strikes in the 1930s, by the 1960s what had been the Morris Motors section was, if anything, the more strike-prone.[16] In this environment, national trade union officials were far less important to most workers than the shop stewards. The attention they received as strikes in the industry became a national political issue in the 1960s may have reinforced this 'oppositional' ethos. There were dissenters, however. There were complaints about the high number of strikes at Cowley, and the Amalgamated Engineering Union and National Union of Vehicle Builders, which both catered for the smaller number of skilled workers, were not always willing to support strikes initiated by the T&GWU shop stewards.[17] Some of the stewards found in both the 1930s and the 1970s that their ambitions went further than those of the workforce. The broader political allegiance to communism or socialism which some of them hoped to develop never emerged.

While this dissenting strand ran throughout the period, one aspect of it remains specific to the 1930s. Then the non-unionism at Morris's contrasted strongly with the flamboyant unionisation at the Pressed Steel factory next door, and it was rooted partly in the ethos of the firm which was still under William Morris's own control, and partly in the native character of the labour force. Drawn from local occupations in which there had been little effective trade unionism, and insulated by generous levels of pay, the Morris workers saw no reason to follow the example set at the neighbouring factory. However, from the 1950s onwards, as the two firms merged with other companies, and labour recruitment ceased to be so representative of Oxford's non-industrial sector, so the roots of dissent going beyond Cowley to a more traditional past ceased to exert much influence. Thus, both the more aggressive shop stewards and the muted opposition which they sometimes faced became if anything more closely tied to Cowley without any involvement in Oxford as the post-war years progressed.

The efforts of the management at British Leyland in the 1970s and 1980s to make the company more profitable required confronting the shop stewards and the fragmented pay systems from which they derived much of their influence. The difficult economic conditions which prompted these measures led to a severe decline in employment at Cowley. Studies of labour in the motor industry in both its aggressive phase in the 1960s and its more defensive posture in the 1980s emphasised its relatively weak links with local communities under both conditions.[18]

College servants, although smaller in number, had a far steadier existence than the car workers. It is difficult to extract a precise number from the census reports because college servants did not have their own category, being returned under general personal service. In 1936 there were 1,140 college servants, in 1988 1,569, the latter looking after a larger number of students.[19] The number of servants who were part-time varied between from college to college, but over time the proportion in any particular college seemed to remain fairly constant. College servants have been portrayed as an especially 'deferential' group, warm to the Conservatives and cool to the trade unions.[20] Some of the changes in their job which did appear to make it less distinctive, such as the increasing burden of summer conference work which was apparent from the 1930s, do not seem to have weakened the strong ethos of the colleges.[21] It was often difficult for servants to move from one college to another, and so dependence on an individual college for earnings was real, and often gratefully acknowledged. At least before the Second World War college employment was highly regarded and much sought after. There is little evidence of any interest in trade unions in the 1930s when they were becoming more prominent locally, nor when the country as a whole was in a more collectivist mood after the Second World War.[22]

Just as there was dissent in Cowley, so there were variations on the prevailing theme in the colleges. While those at the top of the labour movement tended to sneer at the servant mentality of Oxford workers, there were some individuals who proved this to be too simple.[23] If trade unions scarcely made an impact before the 1970s, it is none the less worth noting that H. S. Richardson, a college servant, was chairman of the Oxford City Labour Party in the 1930s, while Arthur Rees, the lodge porter at Wadham College, stood unsuccessfully in two by-elections for Labour in two by-elections in the South ward in the early 1950s. The break with tradition was perhaps clearest in 1972 at St Anne's college with the first strike by college servants.[24] Strikes in sympathy occurred in five other colleges, which gives an idea of the limited spread of trade unionism among the thirty-six colleges in the University. This development owed nothing to Cowley. The earlier efforts to organise the college servants had been made by the T&GWU, the principal beneficiary of the growth of the car works. However, the more successful interest in the college servants in the 1970s came from the National Union of Public Employees.

Between the car works and the colleges lay a number of much smaller enterprises which were closer to the University because of some functional link or because they fitted more easily into the economy of a county town. Some of the firms in engineering and printing were far from small, the University Press employing 840 in 1939, and W. Lucy and Co., an engineering firm, 860 in 1962.[25] The printers had feet in both camps, at the University Press and at the Nuffield Press where they were the exception to non-unionism at Morris Motors before the 1950s. The railway workers were an important traditional working-class group, while those in building were scattered across a number of small firms. Even though many of the workers in these occupations belonged to trade unions, their experiences were very different from those of either the college servants or the car workers. Unionisation amongst the printers and railwaymen was more secure and well-established than at Cowley, and lacked the erratic militancy of shop-floor bargaining characteristic of the motor industry. The printers, railwaymen, and engineers all went on strike in the 1950s but always in response to national decisions and without any particular contribution from local circumstances.[26] While union membership had become a more widely shared experience for many workers by the 1970s compared to what it had been in the 1920s, and had touched even the college servants, it would be a mistake to make too much of this trend to conformity for two reasons. First, the experience of trade unionism varied between occupations and so underwrote rather than weakened divisions; second, while trade unions have been important they are not the only contributors to the working-class outlook.

The role of sport in encouraging mixing between different groups requires assessment. It does seem probable that sport, both as a spectator and participant activity, tended to reinforce rather than dissolve the divisions between occupations with which this chapter is concerned. When the football teams in Oxford were amateur, the pull of a large working-class audience at Cowley was not decisive. Oxford City, the most successful local side before the Second World War, played on a ground to the south of the city and had links with the University which it was unwilling to jeopardise by becoming professional.[27] The other local team, Oxford United, was also amateur before 1945 and played on a number of college grounds against college servants' teams, amongst others. At this level football was reasonably well integrated into the social and sporting life of the old city. However, the growing suburbs of Cowley and Headington gave a greater advantage to a site in East Oxford where Oxford United was located. When this club became professional it drew heavily on the Cowley workers for its supporters. While efforts to secure a ground closer to the car works were fruitless, they none the less provide an accurate indication of the club's source of support. As well as generating an alternative focus of Oxford football away from any influence which the University might have had, the car works also provided successful teams for the local amateur leagues. In the 1920s the Morris Motors team was one of the most successful, and was later joined by those from Pressed Steel. The fact that works teams provided the core of the local football leagues may have strengthened work identities rather than eroded them. The success and strong representation of the teams from the car works may simply have emphasised their importance on the local scene. Likewise, the mixing of students with the town population through sport was limited. There were occasional fixtures with local football teams in the county, and the boys' clubs which were supported by the colleges played those from the town, but there was not the regular participation to match that of the teams from the University Press.[28]

In most respects the students played a small part in the life of the city, even though a significant proportion of them – about 40 per cent – lived in lodgings outside the colleges. Much of their social life took place in the colleges or in the pubs which became strongly identified with them, and most sporting links were inter-collegiate or with teams outside Oxford. The same point – that the town could rarely generate a focus for student energies – was also true for politics. Since the University provided a ready entrée into national politics it is not surprising that the local scene was for the most part ignored. As the trades council complained in 1948, 'ministers can find time, also officials of the TUC, to address members of the University Socialist Club or the Labour Club, but when requested to address a meeting of the Oxford Trades Council this cannot be acceded to'.[29]

Neither labour organisation nor sport overcame differences in geography and employment, but the very scale of the Cowley operation in which some of these differences were rooted was also a dynamic factor encouraging change throughout the city. As Day has noted, the arrival of the motor industry, in offering high wages without the barrier of skill or apprenticeship, altered fundamentally the local structure of employment.[30] Instead of a basic division between skilled and unskilled jobs, where earnings, status, and security were clearly demarcated, the car works offered highly paid if fluctuating employment to many in Oxford, whether they came from the higher-status trades or the less skilled areas. It was never possible for the traditional Oxford businesses to match the wages offered by the motor industry, and so the 'pull' effect was bound to be through individual mobility rather than any trend towards equalisation of pay. While in the inter-war period there was some migration of unemployed labour from the depressed areas, a good deal of recruitment took place from Oxford itself and the surrounding countryside. As the motor industry grew in the post-war years there was every opportunity for movement out of low-paid industrial or service work to higher wages in the car factories. There is evidence pointing to such movements. Those involved in Oxford poor relief in the 1930s found that there was some absorption of labour when the car factories were busy, while the shortage of bus drivers in the 1950s was blamed at least in part on the greater attraction of work at Cowley.[31] Actual disturbance of the job hierarchy was blamed for the decline on status of college work and of the quality of college staff, because of the opportunities for earning more in the car factories.[32] Since there was an expansion of clerical work at Cowley the effect was also noticed in service and clerical jobs in Oxford. Because of the seasonal nature of car production there were also some return journeys, as workers laid off in the summer trough took up building work which was at its seasonal peak. And so even if the collective aspects of Oxford labour reinforced the isolation of Cowley from the rest of Oxford, there is some evidence that individual mobility created a more flexible reality for some Oxford workers.

It is appropriate now to try and investigate degrees of association and transfer in a little more detail. Even if geography and collective organisation suggest segregation, was there still a significant degree of social mixing between Cowley and the 'old' city? Those moved from old housing in the city to new estates on the periphery kept in touch with friends and relations they had left behind; is there any evidence of social mixing without the incentive of earlier neighbourliness?[33] Was the pattern of job mobility different from that of social association, so that there were some transfers but not much mixing? As well as establishing the relationship between Cowley and Oxford it is important to consider what was going on within the longer-established Oxford occupations. Did their status hierarchies remain intact, or did they mix rather more closely as may be imagined for service and industrial workers in a small town?

Evidence with which to answer these questions is not easy to find, and the source used here, Church of England marriage registers, has shortcomings.[34] The problems do not arise from any particular deficiencies in the documents themselves. They provide details of occupations for the groom, the groom's father, the bride's father, and, more erratically, the bride. This material gives a guide as to the sources of labour for particular occupations (groom's and his father's occupations compared) and social association (the same for the groom and bride's father). These details were collected for all marriages taking place in parishes with significant working-class populations: St Barnabas in Jericho, West Oxford, where many printers lived; St Thomas's, to the south-west, wehre many unskilled workers lived; St Clement's and Headington, to the east, which housed a range of service, skilled, and unskilled workers; and Cowley St Mary and St John. From the latter only the marriages involving car-worker grooms were recorded. The chief exception was the parish of St Ebbe's, for which no registers for after 1939 were available for consultation. Usually the certificates give details of occupation rather than the particular firm at which a person worked. However, in the case of car workers, 'Pressed Steel' or 'Morris Motors' was usually entered, which gives a clear demarcation from associated jobs in other firms, which is crucial for pursuing the question of segregation. In a number of cases where a skilled trade was characteristic of the motor industry, for example, patternmaking, this individual was recorded as a car worker.

The small numbers which this material generates might bring reservations about its effectiveness. While there was no sampling within the source, tracing workers through marriage produces a small proportion of the labour force in any particular occupation. It is also the case that there are no figures on occupational distributions by parish, so it is hard to assess if the associations through marriage were more or less strong than might have been expected, given the overall numbers in each occupation. This latter point is not a major problem, since the interest here is in absolute patterns of association or recruitment rather than relative trends. It is the impact of marriage patterns and recruitment paths on different groups which really matters, in the light of residential concentration, rather than such trends with the 'structural' factors abstracted. Those marrying in the Church of England did so in similar proportions as the distribution of social groups in the population as a whole. A large-scale survey using Church of England marriage registers in Oxford showed that the population emerging from the marriage register data corresponded to the population by social class derived from the census.[35] Therefore while marriage registers produce small numbers for any particular occupation, they do not generate a particularly biased sample. They are also valuable source of for historical recruitment to particular jobs, which can only be matched by contemporary enquiries, and these do not exist on any scale for Oxford. Marriage itself is a good guide to family as well as individual association, and by extension, to the mixing between different groups.[36]

The first question to be addressed concerns the car workers: to what extent were they recruited from traditional Oxford occupations, and how did this change over time, so that increasingly those who might have followed their fathers into their jobs (or into other local favourites) went instead to the car works, in search of higher pay? The evidence from the marriage certificates is the reverse of a gradually extending 'draw' upon other Oxford occupations, as the wage signals spread, and as aspirations were modified. Instead, after initial recruitment from a range of occupations, car workers were increasingly self-recruited – sons followed fathers. The first column in Table 6.1 gives the recruitment for the inter-war period, and shows the small proportion (8 per cent) having fathers from the car works with the rest being evenly spread across manual and service occupations.

Table 6.1 *Cowley car workers by father's occupation (%)*

Category	1923–35	1949–65
Car worker	8.5	59.1
Intermediate		
non-manual	6.4	4.8
Service	29.7	9.6
Skilled	28.8	13.2
Unskilled	26.4	13.2
Total = 130		

Source: Cowley St Mary and St John marriage registers, 1923–35, 1949–65.

The second column covers the post war period 1949–65 and shows that a much higher proportion (59 per cent) had fathers from the car factories, with, again, an even, although much smaller spread across manual and service jobs to make up the remainder.

There is no precise correlation with the population of the Cowley parish who were car workers. The nearest figure that is available comes from the analysis of the 1951 census tracts for Oxford by Peter Collison and John Mogey.[37] In the sector which they defined as Cowley (i.e. not the same as the parish) they put 58.7 per cent of the population in the Registrar General's class 3, which would include the majority of car workers, but also any other semi-skilled workers. If anything this suggests a slightly stronger 'self-recruitment' amongst car workers than their share of the working population would have suggested. Elsewhere, the path to the car works was more varied. The only other parish in which there were significant numbers of car workers was St Clement's, which is part of the traditional city, but also in east Oxford. Here, in the post-war period (1946–55), 25 per cent of sons employed at Cowley had fathers there also, roughly half the figure for Cowley.

It is striking that marriage patterns within Cowley suggest even stronger social associations amongst car workers and correspondingly few with those in other jobs. Whereas in the inter-war period 74 per cent of marriages with a car-worker groom involved no other person from the industry, in the post-1949 years the position was reversed: in 87 per cent of car-worker marriages either the bride or the bride's father was employed at either Morris Motors or Pressed Steel. The pattern of recruitment suggests that there had been little disturbance to the labour market in terms of pay and status except in the early years when the car factories were beginning their operations and expanding rapidly. Even then the effect was limited, for most of the new recruits came from low-grade service jobs (gardeners, for example) or from similar occupations; college servants were notably absent as fathers of car workers. After this first decade or so there was a process of concentration. Even more strikingly, the connections which might have been made collectively through trade unions or sport between Cowley and the rest of Oxford seem to have had little or no effect on social associations.

If the car workers seem to have become more separate from the rest of Oxford as time went on, what were the patterns of recruitment and association amongst the other Oxford occupations? College service was a distinctive Oxford job, the attractiveness of which was meant to have declined as conditions within the colleges changed and as the effects of higher pay elsewhere began to make themselves felt. The amount of direct self-recruitment was small as Table 6.2 shows, with only 12 per cent of servants having followed their fathers into college jobs. College servants were drawn from service (chauffeurs, shopkeepers, caretakers) and non-manual occupations (insurance agents, clerks), with a significant number also from skilled trades (joiners, cabinet makers, stonemasons). It is the breadth of recruitment which is perhaps striking. The same holds good for the jobs taken by the sons and daughters of college servants. 61 per cent went into

Table 6.2 *College servants by father's occupation (%)*

Category	1921–60
College servant	12.9
Intermediate non-manual	28.1
Service	15.6
Skilled	25.0
Unskilled	18.7
Total = 32	

Source: St Barnabas marriage registers, 1924–60; St Clement's marriage registers, 1921–39, 1946–55.

the service or non-manual sector, but only 8 per cent went to the car factories. The attractiveness of college employment for a broad slice of recruits from the 'respectable' skilled and non-manual sectors is clear; it is hard to see much evidence of a decline in status in the jobs with which college servants were associated, either in terms of exit or entry. Social association through marriage shows, if anything, a more even-handed relationship between the skilled working class and the service/non-manual groups, with approximately 40 per cent of brides' fathers coming from each. The diffusion of college servants' social contacts in marriage is further emphasised by the fact that in only 13 per cent of marriages in which a servant participated was another servant involved, either as a parent or a partner. Of those employed in printing and bookbinding, 25 per cent had fathers in the same trades; and in 18 per cent of marriages involving a printer or a bookbinder there was another participant from the same trade. Railwaymen showed a stronger degree of self-recruitment than either the college servants or printers, with 35 per cent having fathers in the same occupation. However, even the railwaymen fell far short of the figure of 58 per cent for the car workers, and in general distinctive groups in the Oxford trades did not carve out distinctive patterns in recruitment or association.

The extent to which this was true for broader categories can best be grasped by considering some data on marriage associations by four groupings: intermediate non-manual (clerks, agents, merchants), service occupations (shopkeepers, college servants, butlers, gardeners), skilled workers (joiners, carpenters, printers, railwaymen, upholsterers) and unskilled (labourers, corporation workers, bus drivers). The tables given here for the city parishes provide simply raw data in the form of numbers of grooms' and brides' fathers per category. The figure in the diagonals give the marriages where the groom and the bride's father fall into the same category, and in the majority of cases these are the highest numbers. But the significant number of marriages taking place across these broadly defined groups points to an extensive amount of social association among the Oxford occupations, in contrast to the Cowley experience. Although the grooms from unskilled manual occupations did not marry into the intermediate non-manual category with the same frequency as the skilled workers, they were far from being isolated. They intermarried significantly with skilled workers in of St Clement's and St Barnabas.

Table 6.3   *Association by marriage, St Barnabas, 1924–60*

Groom	Bride's father				
	Intermediate non-manual	*Skilled*	*Unskilled*	*Service*	*Total*
Intermediate non-manual	8	11	5	8	32
Skilled	3	44	32	15	94
Unskilled	4	15	15	7	41
Service	2	8	13	7	30
Total	17	78	65	37	

Given the geographical location of the Cowley suburbs the segregation of their inhabitants from the rest of Oxford, in so far as it is borne out by the marriage data, is not surprising. The Kuchemann survey, which organised the marriage data by social class rather than by specific occupation, found that marital relationships developed over shorter distances as the social scale descended. What the material does suggest is that the potential effect of high earnings at Cowley on the local labour market was offset by other pressures making for segregation. Moreover, while there was a certain hierarchy within the older Oxford trades this did not overcome the close associational interweaving within the particular working-class districts.

Table 6.4   *Association by marriage, St Clement's, 1921–39; 1946–55*

Groom	Bride's father				
	Intermediate non-manual	Skilled	Unskilled	Service	Total
Intermediate non-manual	33	16	9	18	76
Skilled	19	36	21	18	94
Unskilled	9	20	36	8	73
Service	7	12	17	20	56
Total	68	84	83	64	

Table 6.5   *Association by marriage, St Thomas, 1923–59*

Groom	Bride's father				
	Intermediate non-manual	Skilled	Unskilled	Service	Total
Intermediate	11	10	10	7	38
Skilled	9	23	16	6	54
Unskilled	4	9	20	1	34
Service	3	11	6	3	23
Total	27	53	52	17	

At a general level, this chapter suggests that prominent working-class groups in the economy and in the labour movement nationally (in this case the car workers) could live in relative isolation from other working-class groups in the same locality. This same point has significance for Oxford as a university town. The University helped to sustain a certain kind of economy and labour force: it directly employed the college servants and the printers at the University Press, and its custom supported the shopkeepers, builders, and service workers who were also important locally. Even where there was no obvious connection, the character of local industry in its scale and type was in harmony with a university town. Lucy's ironworks in West Oxford complemented the University Press which was located nearby. When Oxford's economic future was being discussed in the 1940s the view that 'one industry which would be welcome in Oxford would be a scientific instrument factory' showed how a certain kind of small-scale industry requiring skilled labour was thought to be appropriate for a university town.[38] The motor industry was not so obviously sympathetic to Oxford's purpose. The degree to which the University was adversely affected can be much exaggerated – Cowley was very separate from the university area, but not so very distant that William Morris was deterred from donating immense sums to the University and colleges.[39] What this essay has shown is that one aspect of Cowley's separation was the lack of disruption of the local labour force to which it had been added and the relative weakness of the connections between them. Local occupations were far from static and unchanging, and those in them did not always correspond to their stereotypes, but many of these changes had little to do with Cowley. The segmentation of the working class left largely unchanged the balance between the University and the local labour force which 'objective conditions' had threatened to alter.

Notes

1   C.J. Day, 'Modern Oxford: economic history', in A. Crossley (ed.), *Victoria County History of Oxfordshire. Volume 4. City of Oxford (VCH)*, London, 1978, p. 218. Day provides a detailed and comprehensive analysis of the local economy.

2   Alan Fox, *A Very late Development. An Autobiography*, Coventry, 1990, p. 13.

3   J. Gottmann, *The Coming of the Transactional City*, MD, 1983, pp. 9–10.

4   See above, pp. 120–2.

5   Letter of city engineer to H.A.L. Fisher of the Oxford Preservation Trust, 8 April 1938, Bodleian Library, Sadler Papers c. 628.

6   E. Ackroyd, 'Retail shops', in A.F.C. Bourdillon (ed.), *Survey of Social Services in the Oxford District*, 1, Oxford, 1938, appendix v, p. 312.

7   Survey of the Cowley Centre in Oxford City Council, *The Cowley Centre*, 1962; D. Murray, *Review of the Development Plan*, Oxford, 1968, p. 69.

8   For the 1920s see R.C. Whiting, *The View from Cowley. The Impact of Industrialization upon Oxford 1918–1939*, Oxford, 1983, p. 40; for the 1970s see R. Taylor, 'The Cowley way of work', *New Society*, 2 May 1973, p. 251.

9   H.W.F. Lydall, 'Liquid asset holdings in Oxford', *Bulletin of the Oxford University Institute of Statistics*, XIV, 1952, pp. 98, 115; 'Personal incomes in Oxford', *Bulletin*, XIII, 1951, p. 388.

10   Material on industrial relations at the Oxford car factories in the 1920s and 1930s is drawn from Whiting, *View*, chs. 2–4.

11 Alan Thornett, *From Militancy to Marxism. A Personal and Political Account of Organising Car Workers*, London, 1987, p. 32.

12 See the efforts of the trades council to enlighten the Pressed Steel workers about the printing strike of 1959. Minutes of the Oxford trades council, 2 and 16 July 1959, held at the Modern Records Centre, University of Warwick, TUC archive, MSS. 292.

13 Steven Tolliday, 'Government, employers and shop floor organisation in the British motor industry 1936–59' in S. Tolliday and J. Zeitlin (eds.), *Shop Floor Bargaining and the State*, Cambridge, 1985, pp. 129–32.

14 D. Marsden *et al.*, *The Car Industry: Labour Relations and Industrial Adjustment*, London, 1985, p. 128.

15 Wayne Lewchuk, *American Technology and the British Vehicle Industry*, Cambridge, 1987, *passim*.

16 Taylor, 'Cowley way of work', p. 251.

17 *Oxford Mail*, 18 August 1959; Oxford trades council minutes, 24 March 1960.

18 H. A. Turner *et al.*, *Labour Relations in the Motor Industry*, London, 1967, p. 165. D. Marsden, *Car Industry*, p. 153. Also Robert Waller, below, p. 183.

19 The figure for 1936 is from *VCH*, p. 220; that for 1988 was supplied to me by Dr Daniel Greenstein, and I am grateful to him for it.

20 See Henry Pelling, *Social Geography of British Elections 1885–1910*, London, 1967, p. 112, and Waller's essay in this volume, p. 181.

21 *VCH*, p. 220.

22 For expressions of gratitude over wage and pension increases (at a time of inflation) see Magdalen College, Bursar's committee minutes, 13 May 1919; for the 1930s, Whiting, *View*, pp. 126–7; for the post-1945 years, 'Unionisation', *Oxford Magazine*, 14 November 1946, p. 78.

23 Whiting, *View*, p. 148.

24 *The Times*, 31 October, 16 November, 8 December 1972.

25 *VCH*, pp. 218–19.

26 For example, the strike in engineering from 25 March to 3 April 1959, and that in printing, which began on 18 June 1959.

27 Useful sources for Oxford football are N. Fishwick, 'Association Football and English Social Life', Oxford Univ. D. Phil. thesis, 1984, subsequently published as *English Football and Society*, Manchester, 1989, and A. and R. Hawkins, *Oxford United*, Derby, 1989.

28 Fixtures reported in the *Oxford Mail*, March, April and May 1959.

29 Trades council minutes, 9 February 1948.

30 *VCH*, p. 220.

31 Trades council minutes, 21 April 1960.

32 J. M. Mogey, *Family and Neighbourhood. Two Studies in Oxford*, Oxford, 1956, pp. 5–6.

33 Mogey, *Family*, p. 83.

34 The analysis is based on marriage registers held in the Oxfordshire County archives for the following parishes: MSS. d.d. Par St Clement's b. 47 (1921–31), b. 48 (1931–39), b. 49 (1946–55), 336 marriages; MSS. d.d. Par St Barnabas, c. 13 (1924–39), c. 14 (1949–60), 216 marriages; MSS. d.d. Par Cowley c. 8 (1923–35), c. 11 (1949–54), c. 12 (1954–58) 296 marriages; MSS. d.d. Par St Thomas c. 14 (1923–59), 198 marriages; MSS. d.d. Par Headington c. 8 (1927–35), b. 19 (1950–58), 102 marriages. The total number of marriages analysed was 1,148 which, since many brides' occupations were not recorded, produced information on the occupations of 3,444 men. A rough guide to the proportion of the labour force emerging in the marriage certificates is given in the table below:

	Nos. employed in 1951	Nos. from registers	%
Car workers	10,000*	401	4.0
Printers	2,310	135	5.8
College servants	1,400	92	6.5

* This is an estimate, to allow for the fact that a sizeable number of the 18,000 car workers employed in 1951 did not live in Oxford. The figure for the college servants is a compromise between the figures for 1936 and 1988 reported in the text.

35 C. F. Kuchemann *et al.*, 'Social class and marital distance in Oxford City', *Annals of Human Biology*, I, 1974, table 1 and p. 17. See also a companion article, 'Social mobility, assortative marriage and their interrelationships with marital distance and age in Oxford City', *Annals*, I, 1974, pp. 211–23.

36 For the use of marriage data in a different context, see Charles Tilly, *The Vendée*, London, 1964, pp. 88–93. An example of a job recruitment investigation is A. L. Bowley, 'The occupations of fathers and their children', *Economica*, II, 1935, pp. 400–7, which dealt with London.

37 P. Collison and J. Mogey, 'Residence and social class in Oxford', *American Journal of Sociology*, LXIV, 1959, p. 601.

38 W. E. van Heywagen, reviewing Thomas Sharp's *Oxford Replanned* in the *Architect's Journal*, 26 February 1948. Cambridge did have such an industry, represented by the Cambridge Instrument Company. On the question of the type of manufacturing thought appropriate for a university town, see Anthony Howe, above p. 21, and Thomas Bender, 'Afterword', in Bender (ed.), *The University and the City. From Medieval Origins to the Present*, Oxford, 1988, p. 292.

39 Between 1926 and 1951 Morris gave £4 million to Oxford University and its colleges. P. W. S. Andrews and Elizabeth Brunner, *Lord Nuffield: A Study in Enterprise and Benevolence*, Oxford, 1955, p. 259, provides a full list.

7 Robert Waller

Oxford politics, 1945 – 1990

In 1945 Oxford University was still represented by two Members of Parliament, while the City of Oxford only returned one, and even this constituency still excluded a considerable part of the urban development to the east occasioned by the boom of the Cowley motor works in the inter-war years. The MP returned in that year of national Labour landslide was a Conservative, Quintin Hogg, the victor of the famous 'appeasement' by-election of 1938. On the city council were still to be found twelve university representatives claiming no party affiliation. Labour did not become the largest party on the council for the first time until 1958, and did not achieve overall control before 1972. The first Labour MP for the city, Evan Luard, was elected in 1966. However, by 1990 the picture was very different. On the city council, now denuded of university councillors and aldermen, Labour held a massive majority with thirty seats to the Conservatives' ten and the Liberal Democrats' five. In parliamentary politics Oxford was now spread over two seats, one of which, Oxford East, returned Andrew Smith, the only Labour MP in the South-East of England outside London. What is more, if the votes within the boundaries of the city had been added up in 1987 it is likely that Labour and Conservative would have been neck and neck – and this in a year when Mrs Thatcher's government was re-elected with an overwhelming majority of over 100! In other words, Labour did very nearly as well in Oxford in their nationally disastrous year of 1987 as they had in their *annus mirabilis* of 1966, and considerably better than they had in 1945, at the beginning of the period under discussion.

How can we explain this relative and absolute improvement in their fortunes, and the apparent decline in Oxford Conservatism?

We shall need to consider not only the course of parliamentary and municipal politics, but the major issues and personalities which dominated the political life of the city over the forty-five years after the end of the Second World War.

In 1945 it is true that Quintin Hogg was fortunate that the pre-war constituency boundaries (in force since 1918)[1] meant that the Cowley and Iffley and the Headington and Marston wards of the city council, which were at that time the chief source of Labour's strength, were still in the county seat of Henley. Had they been included, his Labour opponent, the Hon. Frank Pakenham (later Lord Longford) may well have been able to close the gap of under 3,000 votes by which Hogg retained his seat. Even so, it might be pointed out that Oxford City's 31,625 voters elected one MP, while 15,321 graduates of Oxford University (all with a second vote elsewhere, including many in Oxford itself!) returned two independents, Sir Arthur Salter and A. P. Herbert, and rejected the Labour candidate, economic historian G. D. H. Cole. In 1945 Labour came close to winning both the north Oxfordshire county seat, Banbury, and the south Oxfordshire seat, Henley, than Oxford City.

Even with the 1949 boundary changes which united the county borough of Oxford as a single constituency (and abolished the university seats), Labour did not feel that victory was within their grasp until 1964.[2] There were three parliamentary elections within twenty months in 1950–51; Quintin Hogg defeated Pakenham's wife, Elizabeth, by over 3,500 votes in February 1950, then himself succeeded to the peerage to cause a by-election in November of the same year. The new Conservative candidate, Lawrence Turner, a 42-year-old architect (and nephew of George Grossmith, the actor), never had much difficulty holding the seat during the 1950s; he retired early, reportedly due to business problems, but handed over to the former diplomat and Director General of the Royal Institute of International Affairs, Christopher 'Monty' Woodhouse, in 1959. Woodhouse won a majority of 8,488, or 16.2 per cent of the vote. Oxford City still looked like a safe seat.

Its translation to marginal status occurred between 1959 and 1964. Labour obtained a 6.6 per cent swing from the Conservatives, nearly twice the national average, and well over the figure for the rest of Oxfordshire; only Merseyside seats consistently showed a greater Labour advance in England. Since 1964 no contest in Oxford has been anything other than close-fought (with the possible exception of the inaugural election at Oxford West and Abingdon in 1983).

Table 7.1   *Oxford Parliamentary elections, 1945 – 87*

Election	Electors	T'out	Candidate	Party	Votes	%
1945			Hon. Q. M. Hogg	C	14,314	45.3
			Hon. F. Pakenham	Lab	11,451	36.2
			Wing Cdr F. Norman	L	5,860	18.5
					2,863	9.1
1950*	69,161	84.9	Hon. Q. M. Hogg	C	27,508	46.9
			Lady Pakenham	Lab	23,902	40.7
			D. W. Tweddle	L	6,807*	11.6
			E. Keeling	Com	494*	0.8
					3,606	6.2
			(succession to the Peerage – Viscount Hailsham)			
1950 (2/11)	69,249	69.3	H. F. L. Turner	C	27,583	57.5
			S. K. Lewis	Lab	20,385	42.5
					7,198	15.0
1951	70,494	82.0	H. F. L. Turner	C	32,367	56.0
			G. H. Elvin	Lab	25,427	44.0
					6,940	12.0
1955	67,721	78.2	H. F. L. Turner	C (Ind C) (C)	27,708	52.3
			G. H. Elvin	Lab	19,930	37.6
			I. R. M. Davies	L	5,336*	10.1
					7,778	14.7
1959	66,655	78.9	Hon. C. M. Woodhouse	C	26,798	51.0
			L. N. Anderton	Lab	18,310	34.8
			I. R. M. Davies	L	7,491	14.2
					8,488	16.2
1964	67,011*	77.3	Hon. C. M. Woodhouse	C	22,212	42.9
			D. E. T. Luard	Lab	20,783	40.1
			I. R. M. Davies	L	8,797	17.0
					1,429	2.8

Table 7.1 contd.

Election	Electors	T'out	Candidate	Party	Votes	%
1966	66,303	79.3	D. E. T. Luard	Lab	24,412	46.5
			Hon. C. M. Woodhouse	C	21,987	41.8
			A. D. C. Paterson	L	6,152*	11.7
					2,425	4.7
1970	70,986	74.6	Hon. C. M. Woodhouse	C	24,873	47.0
			D. E. T. Luard	Lab	22,989	43.4
			P. H. Reeves	L	5,103*	9.6
					1,884	3.6
1974 (Feb)	76,645	78.5	Hon. C. M. Woodhouse	C	23,967	39.8
			D. E. T. Luard	Lab	23,146	38.4
			Mrs M. Butler	L	13,094	21.7
					821	1.4
1974 (Oct)	77,270	70.8	D. E. T. Luard	Lab	23,359	42.7
			Hon. C. M. Woodhouse	C	22,323	40.8
			Mrs M. Butler	L	8,374	15.3
			I. Anderson	NF	572	1.0
			Mrs B. Smith	Ind	64	0.1
					1,036	1.9
1979	81,708	74.2	J. Patten	C	27,459	45.3
			D. E. T. Luard	Lab	25,962	42.8
			D. Roaf	L	6,234	10.3
			A. Cheeke	Ox Ecology	887	1.5
			Mrs B. Smith	Ind	72	0.1
					1,497	2.5

Oxford East

Election	Electors	T'out	Candidate	Party	Votes	%
1983	63,613	74.0	S. J. Norris	C	18,808	40.0
			A. D. Smith	Lab	17,541	37.3
			Mrs M. Godden	L/All	10,690	22.7
					1,267	2.7

Table 7.1 contd.

Election	Electors	T'out	Candidate	Party	Votes	%
1987	62,145	79.0	A. D. Smith	Lab	21,103	43.0
			S. J. Norris	C	19,815	40.4
			Mrs M. Godden	L/All	7,648	15.6
			D. Dalton	Grn	441	0.9
			P. Mylvaganam	CC	60	0.1
					1,288	2.6

Oxford West and Abingdon

Election	Electors	T'out	Candidate	Party	Votes	%
1983	67,413	74.0	J. Patten	C	23,778	47.7
			D. E. T. Luard	SDP/All	16,627	33.4
			J. Jacottet	Lab	8,440	16.9
			Ms S. Starmer	Ecol	544	1.1
			R. Jones	Loony	267	0.5
			C. N. Smith	UP	95	0.2
			P. Doubleday	Ind	86	0.2
			Ms R. Pinder	Ind	26	0.1
					7.151	14.3
1987	69,193	78.4	J. Patten	C	25,171	46.4
			C. M. P. Huhne	SDP/All	20,293	37.4
			J. G. Power	Lab	8,108	14.9
			D. Smith	Grn	695	1.3
					4,878	9.0

What happened in the early 1960s? To some extent the unusually large swing was probably connected with the operation of the general factors underlying Labour's advance in Oxford in the post-war period, which will be discussed below, but two factors which might be mentioned in addition here are the inclusion (in 1960) and rapid growth of the Blackbird Leys council estate on the south-eastern edge of the city, and also the great improvement in the organisation of the Labour Party. This was consequent upon the arrival of a new full-time party agent, Harry Cole, and the development of a system of central control of general election campaigns under the energetic supervision of Margaret McCarthy. All wards were now fought in the annual May elections, fully canvassed and leafleted, and special attention was paid to keeping track of those who moved between council houses and of postal voters.³ These efforts were redoubled in 1966 and a further substantial swing elected a 39-year-old academic, Evan Luard, as the first Labour MP for Oxford in 1966.

Oxford now took on many of the characteristics of a 'barometric' or a 'bellwether' seat, usually falling to whichever party won the general elections – it changed hands between the two major parties again in 1970, October 1974, and 1979. In 1983 the Boundary Commission decided that Oxford was too large to remain as a single constituency. They could (as they did elsewhere, for example at Cambridge) have decided to chip off two or three peripheral wards, leaving the core of Oxford intact – this was argued for at the boundary enquiry by some independent individuals led by Nuffield College's renowned psephologist, David Butler. In fact the city was divided into two along the rivers Cherwell and Thames. Oxford East was to be a compact urban unit consisting of the nine city council wards and some other built-up territory east of the river 'across Magdalen Bridge'. The university, city centre, and north, south and west Oxford (six wards) were placed together with Abingdon and several villages in the seat eventually named 'Oxford West and Abingdon'. Both major political parties had reason to be pleased. In place of a single ultra-marginal, it looked as if one fairly safe Conservative and one Labour seat had been created.

In fact, the Conservatives won both Oxford seats in 1983. This was the year which marked the low point of Labour's fortunes nationally, and their campaign was as miserable in Oxford (where the party was bitterly divided and rows about alleged Trotskyist infiltration were at their most severe). The Tory MP for Oxford since 1979, John Patten (formerly a geography Fellow of Hertford College, and rapidly tipped for cabinet office), was returned rather easily in West and Abingdon, and another bright and moderate candidate, Steve Norris, was returned in East by 1,267 votes. It was not until 1987 that Labour came into their 'inheritance', when Andrew Smith entered Parliament, a 36-year-old product of town and gown – a graduate of St John's College who lived in and represented Blackbird Leys, the massive post-war council estate on the edge of the city.

In 1987 John Patten's majority was reduced to under 5,000, but not by Labour. One of the puzzles of Oxford politics since the Second World War is the poor performance of the Liberal Party and their allies and successors at both parliamentary and municipal level.

The Liberals retained their deposit (for achieving over 12.5 per cent of the vote) in only three general elections between 1945 and 1970. No candidate made any real impact, with the possible exception of Ivor Davies in 1959 and 1964; at the age of twenty-three he had dropped out of contesting the 1938 by-election along with Labour in favour of the 'Popular Front' Master of Balliol, A. D. Lindsay. The Liberals were always a distant third in general elections even in a 'liberally' inclined university city, until in 1983 a better prospect was created at Oxford West and Abingdon, which was fought both then and in 1987 by their partners in the Alliance, the Social Democrats. In 1983 the SDP candidate was none other than Evan Luard, the former right-wing Labour MP for Oxford; and in 1987, despite their national decline, the SDP Alliance advanced against Patten with a new candidate, the economics editor of the *Guardian*, Christopher Huhne. There can be little doubt that Oxford's sophisticated electorate indulged in one of the few measurable examples of 'tactical voting'. In West and Abingdon, the SDP Alliance vote went up by 4 per cent and the Labour vote down by 2 per cent. In East the reverse occurred: Labour was ahead by nearly 6 per cent and gained the seat, and the Alliance (here 'Liberal led') declined by over 7 per cent. It is known that Labour shipped many workers, including all those from the University, east of the river, and many voters must have decided to vote against their enemy rather than for their first-choice party.[4] Oxford thus entered the 1990s with two able young MPs, each apparently destined for high rank within their respective parties, both educated at the University and subsequently settlers and local councillors in the city.

Andrew Smith became MP for the bulk of Oxford at a time when Labour were not even close to winning some other seats not too far away, like Swindon and Slough, that they had held in (say) 1959 when the Tory majority in Oxford was nearly 10,000. This relatively strong and improving performance is replicated in municipal politics.

In 1990 the Conservatives in Oxford City Council were reduced to a mere ten seats, and could scarcely be said to form an effective opposition to a dominant Labour group which had been in control for ten years. The Liberal Democrats held five seats, but this was equal to their highest figure since the War on the city council. The Conservatives could not even win control of Oxfordshire County Council, now holding very considerable power over the city's affairs, in 1985 and 1989, and for most important purposes, including the Council budget setting, the county was dominated by Liberal Democrat and Labour councillors. Yet for the vast majority of the period from 1945 to 1980 the Conservatives had effectively run the city council. What accounts for this transformation?

The first thing to be pointed out is that the dramatic shifts in the number of councillors apparent in Table 7.2 have much to do with the well-established fact that a party in national government loses seats in local elections during their periods of mid-term slump. This clearly largely accounts for the Labour decline between 1946 and 1949, when they fell from nineteen seats to five on the council: the rapid Labour recovery between 1951 and 1953 and again between 1956 and 1958; the Conservatives' remarkable advance between 1967 and 1970 and slipping back between 1970 and 1973; and Labour's loss of the council in 1976 and recapture in 1980 and subsequent steady advance.

However, Oxford's council election results do not merely follow the parties' national fortunes. Several purely local factors must be considered. In the first part of our period, up to around 1970, Labour faced various obstacles which made it hard for them to do well on the council, and prevented then from taking control even during Conservative slumps or at their own high-water marks of 1945 and 1966. Three may be picked out.

The first of these was the existence of twelve university representatives, nine councillors and three aldermen, created by the legislation setting up the County Borough of Oxford in 1889 and not abolished till the local government reforms of 1974. Three of the councillors were elected by Convocation (the 'dons' parliament) but the other six were chosen by an even more restricted franchise: the heads and senior bursars of colleges. These nine in turn elected their own aldermen. All were technically independent, but they tended to vote with the Conservatives more often than not, with the exception of one or two inclined to be left of centre, such as the local government expert Bryan Keith-Lucas of Nuffield College.[5] However, their presence did mean that Labour could become the largest elected party, but could not acquire an overall majority, in good years like 1958 and 1966.

The second obstacle was provided by the aldermanic system in general. Between 1945 and 1967 Oxford had 68 members of the council but only 42 of these were elected by the whole adult population

Table 7.2 *Oxford City Council: representation, 1945 – 90*

	C	LAB	L	IND	UNIV
1945	29	19	4	4	12
1946	29	19	5	3	12
1947	36	15	4	1	12
1948	49	5	1		12
1950	50	5	1		12
1951	50	5	1		12
1952	39	17			12
1953	36	20			12
1954	34	22			12
1955	39	17			12
1956	35	21			12
1957	32	24			12
1958	24	32			12
1959	24	32			12
1960	31	25			12
1961	34	22			12
1962	31	21	4		12
1963	27	24	5		12
1964	24	25	5		12
1965	27	28	1		12
1966	29	27			12
1967	37	22			9
1968	46	14			9
1969	51	9			9
1970	46	13			9
1971	36	22	2		9
1972	24	33	1		9
1973	12	30	3		
1976	30	15			
1979	26	19			
1980	21	24			
1982	18	26	1		
1983	15	28	2		
1984	15	27	3		
1986	11	30	4		
1987	11	29	5		
1988	10	30	5		
1990	10	30	5		

of the city. In addition to the 12 university representatives there were 14 aldermen, elected by the city councillors from their own number. The Conservatives used their majority to maintain a quite disproportionate number of their own aldermen for most of the period until the system was reformed in 1974. In 1954, for example, the Conservatives had 21 councillors and 11 aldermen; Labour, with nearly as many councillors, had only 3 aldermen. The consequences was that the Conservatives had fully half of the 68 council members; Labour less than a third. Of course Labour themselves could take advantage of the system when they had the largest number of councillors, but it did have the effect of slowing down change.

Thirdly, there can be no doubt that the ward boundaries were effectively gerrymandered against Labour's interests for the period before 1969. In these years there were seven wards, each returning six councillors (two retiring each year – in November until 1947, then in May from 1949). The wards were not of equal size and became less and less so as Oxford's expansion eastwards continued. In 1951 and 1965, the electorates were as follows:

	1951	*1965*
South	6,880	4,484
North	5,958	5,110
West	6,948	5,083
Summertown and Wolvercote	8,057	8,172
East	10,160	8,328
Headington	14,424	16,310
Cowley and Iffley	16,582	19,072

Labour's strongest wards over the whole period 1945–69 were Headington and Cowley and Iffley. The Conservatives won North every year, often unopposed; Summertown and Wolvercote (in north Oxford) every year except for the Liberal upsurge of 1962, and East and South most years; West was usually Conservative up to the mid-1950s and usually Labour thereafter. By the mid-1960s there were considerably more voters in Headington and Cowley and Iffley wards in outer east Oxford than in all the other five wards put together!

Table 7.3   *Outcome of ward elections, Oxford City Council, 1945 – 68*

	N	S	W	E	S&W	C&I	H
1945	C4	Lab 3 Ind 1	Lab 1 C1	Lab 1 C1	C2	Lab 4	Lab 4
1946	C2	Lab 1 C1	Lab 1 C1	C2	Ind 1 C1	C1 Lab 1	C2
1947	C3	C2		C2	C2	C2	C2	C2
1948	–	–	–	–	–	–	–
1949	C2	C3	C4	L1 C1	C2	C2	C2
1950	C2	C2	C2	C2	C2	Lab 2	C2
1951	C2	C3	C2	C2	C2	C2	Lab 2
1952	C3	Lab 2	Lab 2	C1 Lab 1	C2	Lab 2	Lab 3
1953	C2	C2	C1 Lab 1	C2	C2	Lab 4	Lab 2
1954	–	–	–	–	–	–	–
1955	C2	Lab 2	C2 Lab 1	C2	C2	C2	Lab 2
1956	C2	Lab 2	Lab 2	Lab 1 C1	C2	Lab 2	–
1957	–	Lab 2	Lab 1 C1	C2	C2	Lab 2	Lab 2
1958	C2	Lab 2	Lab 2	C2	C2	Lab 2	Lab 2
1959	C2	Lab 2	Lab 3	C2	C2	Lab 2	Lab 2
1960	C2	C3	Lab 2	C2	C2	C2	C2
1961	C2	C2	Lab 2	C2	C3	Lab 3	C1 Lab 1
1962	C2	C2	Lab 3	L2	L2	Lab 2	Lab 2
1963	C2	C1 Lab 1	Lab 2	L1 C1	C2	Lab 2	Lab 2
1964	C2	C1 Lab 1	Lab 2	C1 Lab 2	C2	Lab 2	Lab 2
1965	C2	C2	Lab 2	C2	C2	Lab 2	C1 Lab 1
1966	C2	C2	Lab 2	C2	C2	Lab 2	Lab 2
1967	C2	C2	C2	C2	C2	C2	C2
1968	C3	C2	C2	C2	C3	C2	C2

Key: N = North   S&W = Summertown and Wolvercote
        S = South   C&I = Cowley and Iffley
        W = West   H   = Headington
        E = East

In 1967, a gesture was made to the continued development of eastern Oxford by the creation of an eighth ward, with just three councillors, Blackbird Leys, which was carved out of the huge Cowley and Iffley ward; these three seats were removed from the university allocation by a Prayer from the city council to Parliament. Then, in 1969, the city council was completely reorganised into fifteen wards, each with three members. South, North and West were so small that they survived with their boundaries almost intact. East was divided into two: St Clement's and a new East. Summertown and Wolvercote became the basis of two new wards (Wolvercote and Cherwell). Headington was split into four (Marston, Headington, Quarry and Wood Farm). Blackbird Leys continued unaltered and Cowley and Iffley was further split in three (Cowley, Iffley and Donnington). The under-representation of east Oxford was over. There were now 30 out of 45 councillors east of the river compared with 18 out of 42 before. The boundaries needed only minor changes in 1979, with the one major exception of the abolition of the Donnington ward and the creation of Central ward, necessitated by the arrival of the student vote in 1970, of which more later. On 1 April 1991 the city boundaries were expanded to include the Old Marston, Risinghurst and Sandhills, and Littlemore wards of South Oxfordshire District, which were already in the Oxford East parliamentary constituency.

Labour's success on the city council in the 1980s was therefore assisted by the removal of the aldermen and university councillors, and by the re-warding of the city, as well as the fact that the Conservatives were in national government for the whole of that decade. However, it is also true that the history of Oxford's electoral politics in the post-war era cannot be divorced from the issues which divided opinion and demanded decisions from the local (and national) politicians. Some of the dominant issues are reflections of concerns faced throughout the country, but many are peculiar to Oxford and require treatment here – although a brief chapter such as this, they cannot be explored in the depth they deserve.

A number of interlinked problems and issues were stimulated by Oxford's geography and provoked complex political responses. The reactions of local politicians to the ideas and proposals of Thomas Sharp provide a fruitful way of examining these. Sharp figures in Oxford's history as a town-planning consultant appointed by the city council in 1945 whose proposals were published in 1948 as *Oxford Replanned*.[7] He also achieved national recognition with his highly popular book *Town Planning* and he was well regarded in the profession for his views on urban preservation. Typically for the 1940s and 1950s, 'preservation' meant a bold philosophy and some brutal solutions. Although Sharp had a warm interest in the countryside he sneered at rustic ornamentation within the city boundaries. He was therefore quite prepared to propose a road through Christ Church Meadow to relieve traffic from the High. To smooth the path of the same road he advocated the bulldozing and relocation of Oxford's working-class neighbourhoods in the south and west of the city.

Table 7.4 *Outcome of ward elections, Oxford City Council, 1969–90*

	1969	1970	1971	1972	1973	1976	1979	1980	1982	1983	1984	1986	1987	1988	1990
Cherwell	C3	C	C	C	C3	C3	C3	C	C	C	C	C	C	C	C
Wolvercote	C3	C	C	C	C3	C3	C3	C	C	C	C	C	C	C	L
North	C3	C	Lab	Lab	Lab 2 C1	C3	C3	C	C	L	L	L	SDP	L2	L
West	C3	Lab	Lab	Lab	Lab 3	Lab 3	Lab 3	Lab	Lab	Lab	Lab	Lab	Lab	Lab	Lab
South	C3	C	L	Lab	Lab 3	C3	Lab 2 C1	Lab	Lab	Lab	Lab	Lab	Lab	Lab	Lab
St Clement's	C3	Lab	Lab	Lab	Lab 2 C1	C3	Lab 2 C1	Lab	Lab	Lab	Lab	Lab	Lab	Lab	Lab
East	C3	C	C	C	L3	C3	C2 Lab 1	Lab	Lab	Lab	Lab	Lab	Lab	Lab	Lab 2
Donnington	C3	Lab	Lab	Lab	Lab 3	Lab 2 C1	C2 Lab 1	Lab	C	Lab	C	Lab	C	Lab	Lab
Iffley	C3	C	Lab	Lab	Lab 3	C2 Lab 1	C2 Lab 1	Lab	Lab	Lab	Lab	Lab	Lab	Lab	Lab
Temple Cowley	C3	Lab	Lab	Lab	Lab 2 C1	C3	Lab	C	C	C	C	L	C	C	Lab
Quarry	C3	C	C	C	C3	C3	C	Lab	Lab	Lab	Lab	Lab	Lab	Lab	Lab
Blackbird Leys	Lab 1	Lab	Lab	Lab	Lab 3	Lab 3	Lab 3	Lab	Lab	C	Lab	Lab	C	Lab	Lab
Headington	C3	Lab	Lab	Lab	Lab 3	C3	C2 Lab 1	Lab	C	C	Lab	Lab	C	Lab	Lab
Marston	C2 Lab 1	Lab	Lab	Lab	Lab 3	Lab 3	Lab 3	Lab	Lab	Lab	Lab	Lab	Lab	Lab	Lab
Wood Farm	C3	Lab	Lab	Lab	Lab 3	Lab 3	Lab 3	Lab	Lab	Lab	Lab	L	Lab	Lab	L
Central	C3	Lab	Lab	Lab	Lab 3	Lab 3	C3	Lab	SDP	L	Lab	L	L	Lab	L

To preserve Oxford's overall identity he also advocated the removal of the motor industry from Cowley. These ideas reflected the unparalleled opportunity for grandiose schemes opened up by postwar reconstruction. More specifically, Sharp himself had connections with the left. Hugh Dalton, who ended up as Minister of Town and Country Planning in 1950–51, had written a foreword to Sharp's study of the Durham coalfield published in 1935, and Dalton's house in Wiltshire, expressing geometric clarity in a rural setting, was used to illustrate Sharp's *Town Planning*.[8]

In Oxford, however, Sharp's ideas were not greeted with unqualified support from the Left. The suggestion that the motor industry be removed from Cowley naturally aroused opposition from trade unionists and local Labour councillors. One of their number, Marcus Lower, did however point out that there was some conflict of loyalty in their protest, because the industrial relocation Sharp proposed was actually consistent with national party policy.[9] The road plan also generated internal divisions. For most of the 1950s the party was in favour of the Meadow road, but five Labour councillors, including Edmund and Olive Gibbs, were expelled from the party's group in December 1959 for voting against it (but both went on to become leaders of that group, Edmund early in 1960, the next year!).[10] It was only in the 1972 election campaign that Labour gained anything from the issue, but this time it was with a policy to reduce the priority given to cars and to avoid the construction of relief roads.

Olive Gibbs again took a leading part in the campaign to defend Jericho in the west of the city from redevelopment in the 1950s.[11] But Labour councillors were not the only defenders of the existing fabric against expansion and change. Conservatives were closely involved in the late 1960s in the protection of North Oxford from the planned university development there,[12] and they too flinched from the efforts of their party's ministers – Duncan Sandys on the need for a relief road and Harold Macmillan over the demolition of the Clarendon Hotel – to plan in Oxford's interests. Overall it is hard to avoid the view that there were councillors from both the Labour and Conservative groups who resisted the efforts to corporate and governmental interests to make Oxford a more pliable environment for growth and change.

Redevelopment is very closely related to housing, one of the most bitter political issues in Oxford in the entire period since 1945. Oxford's geography and, indeed, history meant that there has been a continuous and chronic housing shortage – caused by overtight boundaries, a lack of available land within the city, the large areas of historical interest and space, and the large numbers of students. In 1946 there were 5,000 applicants on the council house waiting list.[13] Between 1945 and 1950 1,400 dwellings were built, but there were still 5,000 names on the waiting list in 1950.[14]

Most of the new housing was in estates several miles from the centre of the city, usually on its eastern edge. Between 1946 and 1977, 1,600 houses were built at Barton. From 1946 onwards 690 were built at Rose Hill (some outside the city boundaries). Between 1951 and 1952 570 were erected at Northway in Marston. From 1953 510 were put up in Wood Farm just inside the eastern ring road. Then in 1957 there commenced the largest development of all, Blackbird Leys, in territory beyond the Cowley motor works transferred from Bullingdon Rural District Council.[15] Three of these estates – Blackbird Leys, Northway and Wood Farm – featured high-rise tower blocks. These were so far away from the city centre that they could hardly be said to impinge on the classic skyline of Oxford, but these peripheral estates offered severe problems of social dislocation – crime, vandalism, youth disaffection, and inadequate leisure facilities.[16]

Despite several other, smaller, council developments within Oxford and estates beyond the city boundaries at Minchery Farm, Littlemore, and Kidlington, the housing shortfall remained acute. This is scarcely surprising in a city which entertained well over 20,000 students by the 1980s: an ever-growing number as the University expanded, and had been joined by a polytechnic, a College of Further Education, and burgeoning of American programmes, crammers and tutorial colleges exploiting the Oxford name. The residential nature of certain parts of the city (such as inner East Oxford) changed from that of a rather conservative, deferential, stable community of college servants and the so-called 'respectable' working class to a predominantly young shifting population of multi-occupiers. Rents were raised and older and local residents pushed out.

There were many battles on the city council over housing policy. Should rent arrears be made up out of city council funds (as Labour usually argued), or should they be financed by higher charges (as most Conservatives believed)? Which party would best be relied on to build more houses? Should council houses be sold to their occupiers, as the Conservatives long held? It was over housing that one leading post-war municipal politician, Fred Ingram of South ward (formerly Labour Agent for most of the Fifties) left the Labour Party in 1960 – he was soon to re-emerge as a Conservative and was to become leader of the council from 1976 to 1980. (Incidentally, Fred Ingram left the Conservative Party in 1983 in protest at the 'extremism' of the Thatcher government and maintains that it is the parties that have changed their position, not he – an interesting point.)[17]

It would be impossible to discuss the major issues in Oxford politics without mentioning education. This is not just because of Oxford's status as a famous university city but because of the battles which have gone on at all other levels of education – from sixth-form provision down to nursery. It was the Conservative council's decision to close down five nursery classes in South and West Oxford which led Olive Gibbs to become politically active for the first time between 1952 and 1953.[18] Oxford's unusual three-tier educational system originated in 1966, when the Labour government issued a circular requiring a plan for a comprehensive system. Labour were effectively in control of the city at that time, and agonised over whether there should be comprehensives for 11- to 18-year-olds or for 11- to 16-year-olds with separate sixth-form colleges. When the Conservatives regained power in the city in 1967 they swept away both ideas in favour of a plan for primary, middle, and upper schools (with internal sixth forms). Labour came back into office in 1972 but this was only a year before the scheme was due to be implemented, so it was accepted and it is still in force.[19]

The Conservatives can count education as one of their most successful local issues, for their system has survived even though there has been continued debate about the three-tier system and also about single-sex education. There are six upper schools in Oxford, two (Oxford Boys and Milham Ford for girls) being single-sex. After the Conservatives lost control in 1985, the county council (in control of education within the city since 1974) decided to merge the two single-sex schools, partly for reasons of rapidly declining rolls – but the Secretary of State for Education refused to allow this.[20]

One issue never far behind the scenes in Oxford concerned the health and future of the motor works at Cowley. Essentially, although there were also fluctuation in the levels of employment there, the post-war era can be divided into two periods: first one of continued growth and boom, as the expansion which had enabled an observer to call Oxford the most prosperous town in England in 1936[21] continued;

then the period of long decline, uncertainty, redundancy, and a slide towards closure. The beginning of the reduction of employment at Cowley came in 1974.[22]

As the war ended, the various motor works (Pressed Steel, Morris Motors, and Osberton Radiators) employed 30 per cent of Oxford's insured population. Far behind came the University Press, and two engineering companies, Lucy's and John Allen and Sons.[23] The motor industry is characterised by mergers, and Cowley was involved in these in both growth and decline: in 1952 Nuffield (of which Morris was a part) joined with Austin to become the British Motor Comapny (BMC). In 1966 Pressed Steel merged with Fisher Ludlow to become Pressed Steel Fisher (PSF), and then PSF together with BMC formed BMH (British Motor Holdings). Two years later the biggest merger of all, BMH with Leyland, created British Leyland. But difficulties dominated the 1970s, and the extent of government subsidy meant that BL was effectively nationalised in 1975. The effect of this major Oxford industry joining the public sector was considerable, as was that of the decline in jobs – from 27,000 at Cowley in 1963 to 20,000 in 1977, as Michael Edwardes began the severe pruning. After the renaming as Rover and the sale to British Aerospace in 1988 the workforce was reduced to only 6,000, more than half not living in Oxford itself by 1990, the year of the McCarthy Committee's gloomy report.[24] It was all a far cry from the new technology of towns like Swindon in the so-called 'M4 corridor' to the south; perhaps Swindon's move towards the Conservatives in the 1980s was not so surprising.

In fact, Oxford's economic base as a whole was hardly likely to lead to great favour being shown to Mrs Thatcher's Conservative government in the 1980s. A declining motor industry, dependent on state subsidy to relieve the threat of unemployment; the great influence of Oxford's health service hospitals at a time when the NHS was seen as the Conservatives' weakest issue of all; the prominence of education, at a time of alleged and perceived government cutbacks, which caused so much resentment in the University at least that the first woman Prime Minister was denied an honorary degree by the dons' 'parliament', Convocation, in 1985. Oxford was indeed relatively good ground for Labour at that time.

It should, though, perhaps be pointed out that the Labour party's latter-day success in Oxford might not all be negative, or based simply on the nature of Oxford's economy. The Labour city council in the 1980s did develop something of a positive reputation as a progressive and active body which (though rates and subsequently the poll tax have always been very high) seemed to offer value for money: certainly there has been energetic self-publicising through events like Fun in the Parks and Oxford in Bloom.[25] The echo of the strongly liberal tone of Oxford's politics recurs. The MP John Patten held that in 1990 the most common theme in his postbag was the environment, threats thereto and the protection thereof.[26] In the May 1990 local elections Oxford was responsible for the highest percentage Green Party vote of any of the 157 local authorities outside London in England and Wales – an average of 11.9 per cent, and three wards in which they were in second place (East, St Clement's and West).[27]

Credit too should be given to the major personalities of Oxford local politics since 1945. One striking aspect is the prominent role played by women in leadership, in all parties. At the end of 1990, nineteen of the forty-five city councillors were female. For the Conservatives, their long-term city council leader was the remarkable Lady Townsend, who had entered the council in 1925 and who remained its leader from 1945 to 1967. Lady Townsend was the aunt of Quintin Hogg, MP for Oxford City until 1950. She was succeeded by another formidable figure, Janet Young, who led the Conservative group from 1967 until after she was ennobled as a life peer by Edward Heath's government on 8 April 1971; she was to be the only woman ever appointed to the Cabinet by Margaret Thatcher (as Leader of the House of Lords, 1981–83). After a short break of male leadership (Bill Simpson and Fred Ingram) the Conservatives returned to their established and successful formula, appointing as head of their group (now in opposition), the doughty Janet Todd of Cherwell ward (1983–91). Among other leading Conservative councillors were (in the 1950s) Alderman Mrs Pritchard and Councillor Mrs Goulton-Constable, and, since 1957, Ann Spokes. In 1990, seven of the ten Conservative city councillors were women. Labour too have had a member of distinguished female politicians.

Until the late 1950s, the Labour group was dominated by a group of right-wing councillors and aldermen based in the Headington ward (which also possessed the popular Labour Club) – Marcus Lower, his wife Florence, Frank Pickstock and R. F. Knight. Both Lower and Pickstock were on the fringes of academic life: Lower was the regional secretary of the Workers' Educational Association (WEA) and Pickstock the secretary of the delagacy of the Extra-Mural Department of the University. Pickstock in particular was a fervent Gaitskellite and a leader of the CDS (Campaign for Democratic Socialism). This placed him in opposition to the dynamic West ward councillor from 1953, Olive Gibbs, who was to become national chairman of CND (Campaign for Nuclear Disarmament) in 1964 and was largely responsible for the move of the Oxford Labour party to a left of centre position in the 1960s and 1970s (much assisted, if often behind the scenes, by her husband Edmund, an accountant and expert organiser). The vital importance of Margaret McCarthy's work, especially at election times, has already been noted.

Another hard-working figure from Headington was Dora Carr, who kept her city council seat in the catastrophic year of 1969, when even Olive Gibbs lost; better known to the general public was the distinctive figure of the Revd Tony Williamson, a worker–priest at Cowley (a fork-lift truck driver) and a Labour councillor from 1961. Tony Williamson and Olive Gibbs were leaders of the Labour group on both the city and the county council for much of the 1960s and 1970s. In the 1980s, the position of the Labour leader had tended to rotate more frequently, with several women playing prominent roles: as the 1990s began, Barbara Gatehouse (Blackbird Leys) gave way to Phyllis Starkey (West ward).

Among the Liberals the party was very much kept alive in North Oxford though the years before the revival of the 1960s by Ivor Davies and Fred Leese.[28] There were sporadic successes in East ward, which elected a sole Liberal, Frankie Powell, to the council in 1949, and provided the parliamentary candidate in both 1974 elections (Margaret Butler, although she had left the party's official lists by 1976 after a disastrous split which led to the loss of all three East ward Liberal seats in the latter year). East ward's Liberalism has been ascribed to various causes, such as the popularity of the East Oxford Liberal Club, but more likely it was due to the anti-socialist, even deferential nature of its working-class vote – traditionally inner east Oxford saw a residential concentration of college servants. The rapid increase of the student vote and the boom of multi-occupation in the 1970s and 1980s have made St Clement's and East safe Labour wards. By the beginning of the 1980s Liberal (Democrat) strength was once again concentrated among academics, in North and Central wards – elected in May 1990 for the latter was the Liberal candidate in East Oxford in 1983 and 1987, Margaret Godden.

The influence of the student vote in the last twenty years is not to be underestimated. Although capable of volatility, like the other sectors of the electorate, in Oxford the student vote has more often than not hurt the Conservatives. It burst upon the scene in 1970. Previously, not only had 18 to 21-year-olds been disfranchised, but the principle of students even over twenty-one having a right to vote in Oxford had been denied on those grounds that they did not live in the city, but were merely visitors.[29] The consequences for local politics were rapidly seen. In 1971, North, which was the only ward in the city which had been universally Conservative since the war, often unopposed, fell to a laboratory assistant standing for Labour, Cyril May. This Labour victory was followed by that of the New College economics don Roger Opie in 1972. The transformation was scarcely surprising, given that the electorate of North ward, which covered most of the colleges (north of the High Street and east of St Giles), nearly doubled from just over 5,000 to 10,000 in the 1970s.

This was to cause the creation of one of the most bizarre electoral units anywhere in Britain. In 1979, the local government boundary commission abolished the smallest ward, Donnington (represented at the time by the Revd Tony Williamson and Andrew Smith, both of whom migrated to Blackbird Leys) and replaced it with Central ward. Central has had an extraordinary political history. Demographically, it is probably the most unusual ward in the nation. Essentially it is completely dominated by the University.

Only 15 per cent of the population was described as 'usually resident' at the time of the 1981 Census. Over 80 per cent of the electorate was aged between eighteen and twenty-five. Eighty per cent was male. Over 90 per cent counted as middle class. For half of the year 80 per cent of the electorate was missing. Approximately 40 per cent changed each year as new students arrived and others left or moved 'into the town'. Of the housing, 3 per cent was owner-occupied, 1 per cent council rented, and over 95 per cent privately rented or college accommodation.[30]

The results this eccentric creature has returned are equally strange. Three Conservatives were selected in its inaugural contest, on General

Election day, May 1979. Within eighteen months they had all vanished, and Labour had made three gains in May 1980 and in a double by-election in early 1981. However, a third brand of politics was also to find favour. In 1982 the SDP won, and in 1983 the Liberals; the decade ended with two Liberal Democrat city councillors in Central ward and one Labour, and the county council seat held comfortably by a Liberal Democrat, the Fellow in Politics at Exeter College, Michael Hart. Six of the ten contests in Central ward in the 1980s had been decided by a single- or double-figure majority.

Even apart from the university councillors before 1974, senior university figures have played a major role in all Oxford parties since the war. As mentioned above, Labour's influential right-wingers of the 1950s, Frank Pickstock and Marcus Lower, were 'fringe' academics. Evan Luard, the first Labour MP, was a Fellow of St Antony's. The University also supplied some of the leaders of the far Left in the party in the 1970s and 1980s, such as the Corpus Christi economist Andrew Glyn.[31] The leading Liberal in Oxford politics from the early 1970s was Dermot Roaf, a Maths Fellow at Exeter College, joined in the 1980s by his college colleague Michael Hart. Among prominent Conservative councillors were John Baker, the Bursar of Jesus (who was Janet Young's father), Robert (later Lord) Blake of Queen's College, John Peach of North ward (a Fellow of Brasenose) – and of course, John Patten, an MP since 1979, a Fellow of Hertford.[32]

The spice of the mixture of town and gown is only one of the fascinating aspects of Oxford city's politics since 1945. In many years it has bucked trends. Starting in 1945 with an entrenched Conservative majority on the council, and with a parliamentary seat that was held by Quintin Hogg even in the very difficult circumstances of 1938 and 1945, it became a classic single-seat marginal between 1964 and 1983, swinging with the tide, and its eastern half elected a Labour MP in 1987 when no other seat did within fifty miles. The 1980s were a period of massive Labour majorities on the city council, which mathematically could not be reversed for some years into the 1990s. The Conservatives even failed to win Oxfordshire County Council in 1985 and 1989.

Some of this move to the left can be put down to the ever present willingness of voters to punish the local election candidates of the government of the day, but this is by no means the whole story.

The nature and economy of Oxford turned it increasingly from Conservatism. Cowley, the great success story of the 1930s and 1950s, became a sick, nationalised, shrinking giant, with the threat of unemployment becoming ever more serious from the early 1970s on. The other bases of the city's economy were no more likely to lead to favour being shown to the Conservative party, particularly Mrs Thatcher's version thereof: the large numbers of health service workers and of those working in all levels of education. The large-scale enfranchisement of students in 1970 did in the end hurt the Conservative Party as much as they may have feared. Demographic changes among the city's residents, particularly in East Oxford, strengthened the hand of the Labour party. Also, the organisation and morale of the city Labour Party improved vastly from the early 1960s onwards, and the Labour administration of the city and Liberal/Labour dominance of the county council proved to the taste of a rather Liberal electorate, much dependent on the public sector, and seeking an active and progressive counterbalance to Thatcherite Conservatism which offered value for money (if not low rates or community charge). In contrast, the local Conservatives often appeared under challenge and on the defensive, able to offer little more than pledges to restrain spending and unnecessary council activity, although the skill and quality of their leadership, predominantly female, should not be underestimated: see for example, their consistent success in maintaining an original and unusual state educational system in the city.

Should Labour win power at a general election in the 1990s, it is likely that the pendulum locally may swing back towards the Conservatives despite the long-term demographic and political factors mentioned above. Cowley may become the site of a battery of optimistic new industries, more suited to the last part of the twentieth century. A national Labour government would be likely to make mistakes that might to some extent alienate Oxford's sophisticated electorate. Oxford remains a competitive political arena, not, thank goodness, a one-party state.

Notes

1   F. W. S. Craig, *Parliamentary Constituency Boundaries 1885–1972*, Chichester, 1972.

2   Interview, Lady (Margaret) McCarthy, Headington, 15 January 1991.

3   Interview, Lady (Margaret) McCarthy.

4   Interview, Olive Gibbs, Oxford, 9 January 1991.

5   Interview, Olive Gibbs.

6   *Oxford Times*, 6 May 1951 and 8 May 1965.

7   *Oxford Replanned*. London, 1948. See also Scargill, above, p. 000.

8   Sharp, *A Derelict Area: a Study of the South-west Durham Coalfield*, London, 1935, and *Town Planning*, Harmondsworth, 1940.

9   Oxford city library, minutes of the Labour party group of councillors, 22 May 1948.

10   *Oxford Times*, 27 May 1960.

11   Interviews, Olive Gibbs and Fred Ingram, Oxford, 16 January 1991.

12   *Oxford Mail*, 7 May 1968.

13   Interview, Andrew Smith, MP, House of Commons, 12 December 1990.

14   C.J. Day, 'Modern Oxford', in Alan Crossley (ed.), *Victoria County History of Oxfordshire. Volume IV. City of Oxford* (*VCH*), London, 1978, p. 207.

15   Day, 'Modern Oxford', p. 207.

16   See, for example, 'Teen trouble at Northway', *Oxford Times*, 17 June 1960.

17   Interview, Fred Ingram.

18   Olive Gibbs, *'Our Olive'. The Autobiography of Olive Gibbs*, Oxford, 1989, pp. 136 – 9.

19   Interviews, Revd Tony Williamson, Forest Hill, 18 January 1991; Dermot Roaf, Oxford, 17 January 1991.

20   Interview, Dermot Roaf.

21   Gilbert, 'Industry of Oxford', *Geographical Journal*, CIX, 1936.

22   Lord McCarthy *et al.*, *The Future of Cowley*, Oxford, 1990, p. 32.

23   *VCH*, p. 208.

24   McCarthy, *Cowley*, pp. 31 – 6.

25   Interview, Councillor Betty Standingford, Oxford, 17 January 1991.

26   Interview, John Patten, MP, Home Office, 14 January 1991.

27   C. Rallings and M. Thrasher, *Local Elections Handbook*, London, 1990, vol. II, pp. 148 – 9, and Table 19 (unpaginated).

28   Interview, Dermot Roaf.

29   See *Oxford Times*, 1 January 1960 (claim of Oliver Impey and others) and *Oxford Times*, 7 May 1971 for Court of Appeal ruling that students can vote where they study.

30   OPCS, 1982 Census, County Ward Monitors, Oxfordshire, p. 4.

31   Interview, Olive Gibbs.

32   Interview, former Councillor John O'Reilly, London, 13 December 1990.

Contributors

Tanis Hinchcliffe is a Canadian architectural historian living in London, and carrying out research on the housing market between the wars. Her book *North Oxford* was published by Yale University Press in 1992.

Anthony Howe is lecturer in international history at the London School of Economics. He is author of *The Textile Masters 1820–1860*, Oxford, 1984, and is preparing a study of free trade and politics, 1840–1914.

Peter Howell is lecturer in the department of classics at Royal Holloway and Bedford New College. He is chairman of the Victorian Society and author of *Victorian Churches*, London, 1968 and was editor with Ian Sutton of *The Faber Guide to Victorian Churches*, London, 1989. He is also a contributor to the forthcoming nineteenth-century volume of *The History of the University of Oxford*.

Elizabeth Peretz is completing a doctoral thesis on maternal and child welfare between the wars and was formerly a research assistant at the Wellcome Unit for the History of Medicine at Oxford. She contributed to Jo Garcia, Robert Kilpatrick, and Martin Richards (eds.), *The Politics of Maternity Care: Services for Childbearing Women in Twentieth Century Britain*, Oxford, 1990.

Ian Scargill is a fellow of St Edmund Hall and lecturer in geography in the University of Oxford. He is author of *Urban France*, London, 1983, as well as many essays on Oxford and the surrounding region.

Robert Waller is research director at The Harris Research Centre. He is author of *The Dukeries Transformed*, Oxford, 1983, and *The Almanac of British Politics*, 4th edn, London, 1991.

R. C. Whiting is senior lecturer in history, University of Leeds, and author of *The View from Cowley. The Impact of Industrialization upon Oxford 1918 – 1939*, Oxford, 1983.

Index